Bubble Gum Badge

Bubble Gum Badge

An FDA His-Story

Patrick Stone

Library of Congress Control Number: 2011907752
ISBN: Hardcover   978-1-4628-7259-6
                 Softcover   978-1-4628-7258-9
                 Ebook   978-1-4628-7260-2

Print information available on the last page.

Rev. date: 06/12/2014

To order additional copies of this book, contact:
Xlibris
1-888-795-4274
www.Xlibris.com
Orders@Xlibris.com
591621

Contents

I dedicate this book to the FDA investigators in the field, support staff, lab staff, and the Reviewers in FDA Headquarter Divisions. Without your work and sacrifice, our country would not be as safe, and our health products would not be among the most effective. Thank you to my colleagues, friends, and family for putting up with my antics and big head!

Before I decided to resign my position with the FDA, I followed the chain of command for grievance, and wrote a final letter to the commissioner and secretary of HHS. This final communication with upper management provided my thoughts for reducing agency waste and mis/micromanagement issues. In my mind, I only needed a reason for hope, just one word! Unfortunately, I did not receive a reply or intervention.

I turned in my gold FDA badge and walked away, hoping to still be of service to our global health because I am duty bound. A desire for global health infects your inner soul and requires one to be of service to our nation's health. I still proudly wear my ten-year US government bronze service lapel pin because I swore an oath to protect the US (and global) public and I have not renounced that oath or relinquished my sworn honor to protect our global health market.

Without passion for what drives mankind to achieve a seemingly impossible challenge (such as global health) our legacy will be lost in ashes. If I can help your health product on its life cycle to market, please contact me at the links below.

Email: *Patrick@tradestoneqa.com*
Web-site: *http://www.tradestoneqa.com/*

PREFACE

A FEW YEARS ago, I put together a collection of my thoughts regarding the US FDA and my personal experiences over 13 years as a field investigator in Texas. Since then I have had the opportunity to experience a world of new opportunities as a consultant, so I thought it was time to revisit the Bubblegum Badge world. Along with a few colleagues, I have added several new sections and have tightened up some of the language and phrasing. It is, as with everything in life, still a work in progress . . . .

As I said in the first edition of this book, I don't intend this book to be either a roasting or a toasting. I hope what it will do is provide a glimpse of what the FDA does well, and what it needs to improve on (as evidenced by audit reports from the Health and Human Services [HHS] Office of Inspector General [OIG]).

The name "Bubble Gum Badge," by no means suggests a weak or ineffective organization, rather, it is something my friend from the Imports Division stated during a happy hour we were at in 1999. He put it this way: "If you think that gold FDA badge is going to get you out of trouble, son, you are wrong! It's a Bubble Gum Badge and is more trouble than you have ever known." Thankfully, I did not get into any real trouble as a young man with a great responsibility to protect and serve. There are many ways to keep harmful products from the US market, and some of which take longer than the proverbial slow boat to China. I was a frontline grunt out in the field, conducting the FDA business of the day. Those twelve years and eight months were some of the most challenging and rewarding moments any one person could ask for.

When you sit down to eat today or see your family member take their medications or go into surgery, you can rest assured that *at least* one of the FDA's finest had at some point in the product's life cycle taken a look to see if it passed inspection. FDA does the work that is most taken for granted and expected as a given by the US public. Your tax dollars were always hard at work when I was on the job, even though it may not have always appeared that way.

I would like to thank the FDA for taking me around the world and giving me the best training anyone can ask for in this quality assurance (QA) business (on-the-job training). FDA needs your help and more regulatory authority for biologics, drugs, and devices. Only Congress can grant more FDA authority, and budget battles seem to be the mainstay. Most of the information I reference comes from the public domain site www.fda.gov. The FDA's mission is too important not to be modernized, supported, and innovated. FDA falling behind in modernization would mean lives at risk globally.

The oversight of our global health market is waiting. If you want it and qualify, your official gold FDA badge is waiting for you. FDA has mine in a vault next to my government international passport (I have my old decommissioned one). Anyone reading this book can be an FDA Consumer-safety officer (CSO)/investigator. Trust me when I say sixty semester hours of accredited college science and some luck on the computer lottery (usaJobs.opm.gov) and you're in. I would suggest higher than a Bachelor of Science education for entry into bioresearch monitoring. As an ex-FDA recruiter and mentor to many new hire FDA field investigators, I would say a graduate degree or higher also assures your entry to drug and device program field work.

So, take a look behind the kitchen, Pharmacy, and hospital operation-room doors with me. Thank you, global health providers and professionals (all of you)! Thank you, health-care receivers, all of you; without you, there would be no need for health-care products. I think that includes everyone in the world!

Thank you for your time and for coming along to take a microscopic view into one of the most unsung agencies. FDA has very little glitz or glamour and I hope you find something you find interesting in this book.

CHAPTER 1

The Journey begins

MY JOURNEY AS a field investigator with FDA (also known as a Consumer-safety officer (CSO) or investigator) began in August 1998 with the swearing of an oath and a badge and credentials presentation. My supervisory Consumer-safety officer (SCSO) at the time was a thirty-year veteran with military war service. He had, literally, seen it all, and knew which of us would contribute and which of us would fold under the weight that came with the FDA mission. He read us the riot act and the FDA preamble, and warned of credential misconduct; he also warned us that "immoral acts" (and/or the appearance of impropriety) were enough to terminate a new hire during the one-year probationary period (two years, if you were considered career-conditional). Many of the forty newbies in my hire class left the FDA or the Dallas District within the first three years of service.

When I transferred to the Austin Resident post in 2010 in the shadow of the burned-out Echelon I building (just after a Mr. Joseph Andrew Stack flew his plane into the IRS building,) I hoped it would be better than the two major hurricanes I left behind in Houston. No such luck! No one flew a plane into us, but we had just as many anonymous callers harassing us and complaining about FDA work as we got in Houston. Folks, the grunts in the field do what US Congress and the commissioner tell us! Call your US congressman to effect change or enter your issues into the FDA Facebook page, please! The field investigators do not have any control over what FDA decides is necessary for the public health. That is all I will say for security matters. I will abide by the rules for protection of individually identifiable health information.

I will not mention subjects or studies I have investigated. This book is about our future and present mission as global health providers. Privacy Laws and Health Insurance Portability and Accountability Act (HIPAA) rules will be followed. Neither sponsors nor corporations of any nation will be referenced. I will mention a few of the national health organizations that we all have access to on the World Wide Web (Argentina, Brazil, Canada, and European Medicines Agency). I have worked with these organizations during official FDA international inspections, and I encourage you to fact-check your request through the Freedom of Information (FOI) Act my investigation reports. (I will forewarn you, FDA mandates the report template and content, so they are a little dry as in robotic; but the facts are there.) My official training records and contact information are provided in the back of this book. I hope to be of service to your clinical trials and Global Health product Initiatives.

I am not by any means knowledgeable about all things FDA and only know a little bit about a few different program areas. I do not speak for the FDA nor have I ever spoken for the FDA. I was never granted the authority to give an official government approved interview or speak on behalf of the agency. I have given presentations to industry on behalf of FDA Dallas District management, but these were not in a mass media forum. The FDA has not endorsed or provided me with official comments for this manuscript. My opinions are simply my personal, free expressions of speech formulated through years of regulatory experience.

I am not a disgruntled employee either; I have nothing but respect for the field investigators, laboratory staff, support staff, and frontline fieldworkers; as well as the center reviewers. I just observed so many areas where agency or government change could have been effective in saving tax dollars, being earth friendly and efficient. I made many suggestions, and proposed pilot programs to cross-train Review Division and field investigators for operational awareness to no avail. I also put forward paperless program requests and recycling eco-minded initiatives. I tried to inject logic and scientific method with little or no tangible results. It was like, "There goes Stone again trying to be an Eco-ranger, what a joker." I was not joking, and sustainability is not a joke either. I gave it my best and even commuted between Houston and Austin twice every week for four years to keep on serving. In the end, I simply could not comply with orders sidelining my BIMO work. FDA must conduct more BIMO to pay the bills and for public health (user fee act monies). One percent FDA domestic clinical trial review may not always ensure public safety. No hard feelings on my part, I just hoped for the better with documented scientific results, not political blather.

The training for FDA field personnel was mostly on-the job. It's a little scary when you think about it – the very personnel impacting products and public health get little formal training before they are let loose into the field. The FDA training was not centralized or done by the Office of Regulatory Affairs University (ORAU) when I started in 1998. The ORAU was founded around 2003, and much of the investigator training is currently done online or in Washington DC at the Rockville ORAU campus. (Basic law and persuasion techniques (information gathering) for us were conducted in Jacksonville, Florida, in 1999, and we had a blast forming unit cohesion. I keep in contact with more than a few of my fellow basic training crew.) The ORAU does not seem to be able to keep up with the current demand for state and federal investigator training as new hire roles increase. The FDA is asked to do a titan's job, training new hires and seasoned field investigators. Training for the health products FDA regulates is neither easy nor quick, and product approval time is measured in decades. The FDA regulates approximately 95% of the goods and services we use daily (lasers, microwaves, plates, flatware, food, drugs, medical devices, blood and multispecies biological products, food and drug imports, etc.) with very little regulatory authority for timely consumer protection action.

CHAPTER 2

Food Work

MOST FDA NEWBIES start out in food work, and we were hired under the implementation of the Food Safety Initiative (FSI) Seafood Hazard Analysis of Critical Control Points (HACCP) regulations, which resulted in the formation of the Office of Seafood. I feel it is important to start here so you understand that most FDA investigators start conducting food program work. The FDA requires investigators to learn title 21 of the Code of Federal Regulations (CFR) and food laws pertaining to the established precedents. Each new hire learns the basics and works their way to their desired program area or the program area selected for them by their supervisor. We all learned the seafood HACCP inspection techniques in March 1999, and by April 1999, all eight of us new hires in the Houston resident port were conducting numerous solo shrimp and finfish Seafood HACCP inspections.

FDA does not check the restaurants you are eating at. Your local county or city health inspector performs this task. Rather, FDA regulates food commodities that enter into interstate commerce. What that means is that if your processed or unprocessed food product crosses a state-line, FDA or USDA will inspect your place of business/firm (warehouses, manufacturing plants, etc.). Would you believe that prior to 2011, FDA could not easily compel or order removal or recall of foods from the market? This has changed since the Food Safety Modernization Act of 2011(FSMA.) The FSMA grants the Foods Division recall authority and enhanced food-regulation authority for the FDA, the focus being seafood and products eaten raw (veggies, fish, milk, etc.). The big problem right now for the FDA is funding and allocation of resources (logistics).

The current consolidation effort to bring all centers (biologics, drug, device, and food) and departments in one campus will be a great benefit and a great expense, all in one package. Newly constructed buildings at White Oak will replace all the existing fragmented facilities which support the Office of the Commissioner (OC), the Office of Regulatory Affairs (ORA), the Center for Drug Evaluation and Research (CDER), the Center for Devices and Radiological Health (CDRH), the Center for Biologics Evaluation and Research (CBER) and offices for the Center for Veterinary Medicine (CVM). The development will consist of new laboratories, office buildings and support facilities. This consolidation project has been authorized through the FDA Revitalization Act and is funded through the GSA appropriation.

The FDA's current information technology (IT) modernization process is about five years delayed, and IT product procurement is outdated. The new mandatory security measures for employees and IT are also new major expenses. Training is always one of the first cut programs and most vital to seasoned investigators and new hires alike. The Office of Regulatory Affairs University does what it can; however, the ever-increasing need to contract state inspectors to conduct FDA work training must be provided by the state inspectors. Food training is taking precedence with food-safety monies, and other center trainings (CBER, CDER, and CDRH) have taken a backseat. All hands on deck for food work with congressional mandates, regional performance, goal work, and international inspections. Video link systems, already in every office, can be used for training and may help alleviate this issue. All the different centers have quarterly telephone meetings, but very rarely are the video links used, other than for all hands-on regional district meetings. With fuel and energy costs rising, innovative efforts will have to be implemented to train this new crop of investigators.

FDA is in business to keep the US public safe. At what point does it make it right for the FDA to steer the domestic market and food production in a certain direction with laws that infringe on free-market ideals? The markets (small businesses and large corporations) should choose their own path and not be dictated as to the choices of safe food and health-care products to be offered at market. FDA needs to regulate food labeling so that genetically modified organisms (GMO) and products made from GMOs are fully labeled at your food market. Labeling should also state if any component of that food product is an import (quantity percent included). We need to know what we are eating and where it is from. Is that really too much to ask from the food manufacturers? After all, we are in the great age of information and transparency. We do have some domestic food producing "bad apples"; however, most food-borne illness outbreaks come from imported products (gray/sewage water used on vegetable crops, insect contamination, radiation, dioxin, pesticides, and many other toxins) or deal with product the USDA should handle but defers to FDA.

The USDA has two times the amount of inspection staff yet defers most USDA recall work to the FDA Center for Food Safety and Applied Nutrition (CFSAN). USDA usually defers any of its recalled products because the USDA inspectors are not as familiar with recall checklist procedure. The recall audit-check list is literally a checklist and telephone call-based audit form or personal visit. In many cases, the audit checklist can be accomplished by any college grad. The audit-check recall-form questions establish where the product was purchased, lot information, storage information, the quantity of product in stock, manufacturer ship back information (for product destruction/reconditioning), address and telephone information, customer complaints, customer illness, and finally, how the seller was informed about the recall (e.g., letter, fax, or phone call). You tell me if this sounds so difficult to accomplish. I will stand corrected if you feel I am burdening USDA inspectors with too much science.

I have read many recent US government reports stating there is too much overlap of food regulation and inspection, and it should be paired down to work in conjunction with all food-inspection agencies. I will only believe that when I see it because it would be a first and could be classified as a miracle. An excerpt from "Oversight of Food Safety Activities: Federal Agencies Should Pursue Opportunities to Reduce Overlap and Better Leverage Resources" Government Accountability Office (GAO-05-213, 2005) reports the following: "GAO has documented many problems resulting from the fragmented nature of the federal food safety system and recommended fundamental restructuring to ensure the effective use of scarce government resources. In this report, GAO (1) identified overlaps in food safety activities at USDA, FDA, EPA, and NMFS; (2) analyzed the extent to which the agencies use interagency agreements to leverage resources; and (3) obtained the views of stakeholders" (*http://www.gao.gov/products/GAO-05-213*). The Center for Food and Applied Nutrition has on numerous occasions testified to Congress that food-inspection overlap is an incorrect assessment of the partnership among multiple US government agencies.

This report appeared in May 17, 2005, in "The Subcommittee on the Federal Workforce and Agency Organization House Committee on Government Reform" (*http://www.fda.gov/newsevents/testimony/ucm112947.htm*).

The food-inspection overlap is apparent especially when you consider county and state inspections on the heels of FDA food inspections. The FDA currently contracts thousands of food inspections each year to state-counterpart agencies and trained state auditors to conduct FDA-regulated industry. The FDA also routinely observes state inspectors on food inspections for training and verification purposes.

The FDA training regimen is constantly evolving and fluid in nature. In 1999, we started with the Seafood Hazard Analysis of Critical Control Point (HACCP) regulator training, food and drug law, and the Seafood HACCP encore training. The Seafood HACCP encore training was basically a refresher course because most of us had a hard time grasping the HACCP concept through the Seafood HACCP guide. In 2001, a new, improved guide was put out to help us better understand the seafood guide and to correct glaring scientific errors in our HACCP field guidebook. By 2002, we were given another Seafood HACCP training, the trainer encore class to help us explain the regulations to the international shrimp harvesters with very little English skills or fishing-focused business minds. With the gulf oil spill, their livelihood is at risk even more so now with the miles of documented oxygen-depleted dead zones and red tide blooms. Most of the seafood hazards are man induced, such as allergens in sodium bisulfite agents or time temperature abuse. Modified atmospheric packaging has become a very hot FDA food topic. The issue is simple: keep your product frozen and there is no acute bacterial hazard other than slow-growing, cold-tolerant bacteria. There is very little glory or big cases in the food industry, but that does not stop the FDA from trying. Warehouses and interstate-trade food producers rarely have intentional misbranding or lethal human intent. Luck of the draw is usually how you encounter a very big food case that has state, national, or global implications (melamine, antibiotics, or other harmful toxins).

Large food warehouses are always a problem when not maintained properly, and many sources of contamination can enter the market through these firms. Most of the work on the Gulf of Mexico coast in the Houston area is on shrimp harvesting and processing, blue crab processing, and shellfish (oysters and mollusks) harvesting. Many of us did the same firm inspections for three or four years. I especially enjoyed going to South Padre Island, Texas, for the shrimping season and two-week inspections; it was really rough duty. I also always enjoyed going to see the alligator processors and the big gators they would harvest during the alligator-hunting season.

The alligators hauled in are usually bigger than the boats that bring them in. (A thirteen-foot, twelve-hundred-pound gator laid out in front of you is an awesome sight, knowing it was harvested not too far from the processing-dock bayou.) I like seafood, and I think it is very important to a balanced diet; however, man-made influences have diminished the Gulf of Mexico seafood stocks and those of the world. I am very cautious when purchasing seafood at the local food market. I always check the seafood harvest area since the Japanese Pacific Ocean radiation event and the BP spill. Radiation contamination will now also be a great concern to those of us who see stories like the tragedy of the Japanese Fukushima Daiichi Nuclear Power Plant contaminating the Pacific Ocean.

Some of the investigators went to work in devices, drugs, and biologics programs. Many new hires stayed in the food inspection area, 75 percent of our FSIS group (approximately). I conducted an average of twenty seafood inspections in addition to fifteen bioresearch monitoring (BIMO) from 2000 through 2002. In 2001, I changed supervisors because there were too many of us for one person to manage in the Houston office. My next supervisor was very knowledgeable about FDA and had twenty-plus years in grade. She hesitantly fostered my BIMO career, making sure I still did food sampling, drug, and food work. She was a BIMO field investigator and knew that a strong foundation on FDA basics made a great BIMO investigator. She kept me grounded and then flew me off into the international travel arena. She also fostered my extracurricular FDA activities like the Dallas District Hispanic Employee Program Representative (HEPR). The HEPR is responsible for recruiting and maintaining Hispanic workforce in the FDA Dallas District (Texas, Oklahoma, and Arkansas).

I hosted educational events for Hispanic Heritage Month in the FDA office and off site and provided mentorship for George I. Sanchez Charter High School students and college students in the Greater Houston, Texas, area. I also presented and gave talks at local universities for college students about what FDA does for a living. I still recommend FDA to any scientist that wants to make a global difference as a career choice. FDA can take you to the four corners, but you have to get in there and get to work, or you will just be a desk jockey watching your colleagues shoot off into the stratosphere. I was awarded many national FDA accommodations as a direct result of the training and encouragement from my first two supervisors.

Sampling human-food commodities is one of the basic functions we all endure. Whether it's an imported food product (from every continent and nation) or domestic (homemade, born in USA) food, we collect it. The port of Houston is the third biggest coast in the nation, and Houston receives more cargo by boat, train, plane, and highway transport than the entire border of Texas combined.

The border in 1998 at each Texas border town of entry (main NAFTA bridges) was staffed with at least six investigators. The funny thing for me or scariest, and I am not afraid of much, was that in 1998, there were three import investigators covering the whole Houston port of entry. I remember seeing my buddies' desk filled to the ceiling, high with documents for imports, products awaiting clearance for entry into Houston supermarkets/local markets. Now 2011, they have a large staff of twenty or so investigators plus the behind-the-scenes import coverage with homeland security/customs border patrol, etc. I could not believe with my own eyes how FDA looked (physically sampled or looked at other than a computer screen) at less than 1 percent of the imported goods incoming from every nation to the port that is Houston in 1998. The import division does have its problems, but that is for another book by another expert. I will not pretend to know how exponentially more imports there are to clear, but I know it is more than current staff can handle. The Imports Division needs experienced and knowledgeable management in the field that can balance market safety and political hot air.

I can only tell you that my family buys and eats mainly food from Texas or naturally harvested seafood. Do some research on our current salmon aquaculture methods and you will see we have a long way to go before proceeding responsibly. I have seen aquaculture farms for certain crustacean (shrimp and crawfish) species not using antibiotics and using water-friendly and earth-friendly methods of production. Antibiotics, pest species, and chemically enriched pellet food are endangering native species and the water supply. Many aquaculture fish stocks are genetically modified fish, which then escape the farm and breed into the native species (approximately 3%; 1 fish is too many). We are playing god, and yes, we have great knowledge on how to splice genes and use bacterial and viral vectors to change DNA in order to make new species. However, the research scientists are just now unraveling the protein-folding kinetic mystery. There is much to learn about prion proteins and protein-activation signals. Who knows what is being "cooked up" out there in dark laboratories?

When you talk about the molecular and genetic level of our current capabilities, we are still second generation. It is like we are looking into space with a telescope and all we see are old pictures of the stars' light. I am trying to convey urgency because this scientific field has a lot to learn about the so-called empty or blank regions of the genetic code and how generations of xenomorphic (plant genes comingled with animal, bacterial or viral-vector-transfected hybrid species) species will interact with our native species. I am all for autologous (self) cells from one's own body or interspecies (at least mammalian) health treatments, but the outright genetically changing of food into "Frankenfood" so it can grow faster or devour natural resources without regard to the following generations or other competing species is ethically wrong in my opinion. Duke has a very challenging case study on this subject (*http://www.duke.edu/web/kenanethics/CaseStudies/FDA.pdf*).

Our Native American brothers have been right the whole time. We must live responsibly and treat the earth with respect, or the earth will expel us and start over as it has many times in the earth's life cycle (I digress). I am not in any way trying to persuade you in any direction. I am trying to present facts and discussion points. You all must choose what you and your family consume for health and body energy. We live in a free society with a free market; let's keep it that way. We are not perfect, and we never will be. Perfection is our diverse cultures working together to achieve global health and future sustainability. No one nation can provide total public health; it is a cooperation in effective symbiotic harmonization. Effective organizations respect partners with novel approach strategy and incorporate effective solutions to global health problems. Using what works and discarding what does not work is an evolution process, which must be allowed. Discarding failed ideas is a natural part of the scientific method.

On the domestic (in the US) side of FDA, we learned to sample local-grown corn for aflatoxin (very toxic fungus that grows on corn), farm-animal feed, seafood, fresh produce from large warehouses, over-the-counter drugs, dietary supplements, and everything in between. I was so sampled out by 2004 that only doing bioresearch monitoring was a good change of pace. Sampling is a very important part of food vigilance for consumer protection.

FDA expends a lot of manpower and resources to make sure at least 1 percent of the local commodities are sampled for market safety. FDA relies heavily on state counterparts and city and county health departments for enhancing sampling and food-safety vigilance. FDA, in many cases, pays for the samples it tests in many of the food laboratories around the country. During the FDA reorganization and modernization efforts, many laboratories were on the chopping block, and most of the investigators in the field could not believe that FDA would close labs that were overloaded with samples and could barely keep up with what we sent to them. Anything FDA needed to modernize; the current laboratories spent some funds on much-needed modern test equipment LC/MS/MS mass spectrometry, and highly accurate bacterial and viral testing equipment and maybe even some sensitive equipment to check for radiation. Congress quickly stopped the closure of any much-needed laboratory and staff members. Many laboratory folks left the agency or moved to domestic investigations only to find out the laboratories were here to stay and maybe get some retrofitting and upgrades. In my opinion, FDA and the CDC should apply for national/congressional grants to procure or acquire prion-protein-detection equipment and test methods.

I do think Congress should have cut the handful of regional directors and upper-middle management staff because in the end, they go to meeting after meeting to make sure the beans are counted (computers can accomplish this for free). FDA needs those funds to acquire more worker bees (investigators and product-review division staff). Does FDA really want to break new records in physical food and drug product inspection (not including paper review or online, which is much higher)? If so, then FDA needs more working manpower for all departments and divisions.

FDA has almost as many "Chiefs" as it does "Indians." Please pardon my analogy – I am part Native American and use this analogy often. FDA is seriously understaffed and has more work to do than can be done with what is available. I will use the Houston resident post as a measuring stick to illustrate how FDA conducts the business of the day. The average resident-post size was fifteen domestic investigators and two support staff (office assistant level), who copied reams of paper and mailed off tons of reports. Without the support crew, Houston would have never got the job done. Houston traditionally always met the district goal numbers and congressional mandates, so I was always proud of that fact, at least. Most of the crew pulled their weight, but we are all human, and the bell curve applies with government workers. The Austin post had four investigators and no in office support staff. It did take me extra (30 percent) administrative time to package the report submission, and I missed my administrative support staff. You have very good people that do the work of two, and those that do half day's work on a good day and nothing on Friday. Of the fourteen investigators, five were dedicated to food work, two for device work, two for drug work (with me as backup), three for biologics, and two for bioresearch monitoring. The drug, device, and biologics people overlapped into other program areas; and food sampling was around at least 10 percent. So you can see we were spread very thinly. The Greater Houston area population at present is close to six million individuals.

When you talk about food production in our post-9/11 world, you must mention bioterrorism over watch, enhanced sampling, and cooperation from regulated food industry. A reasonable tone with plain language is necessary for regulated industry cooperation and partnership. FDA still needs to learn the art of plain language and quit the old "barking-out-orders" routine; it will simply not work. FDA is responsible for bioterrorism/pandemic response and many other very serious matters that must not be diluted by the micromanaging of the food area. In 1998, we did not sign up to be called bioterrorism and pandemic responders, but answered the call and stood at the ready. I want to give thanks to our volunteer military and civil servants, many of whom go to the FDA to complete their lifelong public service. Thank you again to all our US volunteer armed forces for your sacrifice to defend our freedom of choice and speech. I also want to thank those service men, women, and canine that have given the ultimate sacrifice for our way of life.

Farmers and the small-business sector make this country great, and FDA should not be squashing this sector of business in the name of security, or we will not have anyone to protect. In 2002, the whole way FDA looked at incoming food product and domestic production changed forever. FDA is requesting food producers to provide documented histories of every worker. FDA needs to know if you conducted background checks and acquired legal status checks of workers to work in the United States. We are vulnerable in the food arena, but we should not treat our domestic producers as guilty before proven innocent. Look at the recent actions regarding raw milk and milk products. I am not sure that unarmed Amish and Quakers or anyone selling unpasteurized milk and cheese should be taken down with guns at the ready. These are Americans trying to make a living. FDA should educate food producers or show positive proof that adverse events/deaths have occurred from their firm's product before going in with guns blazing. I understood and did my duty when individuals knowingly caused harm or, by acute negligence, caused harm to another human. At times, I feel ashamed to be ex-FDA with the type of perceived overkill for the producers of these milk products.

The burden of proof is on the government to show willful harm to the public. I have not seen the bodies stacking up from individuals drinking unpasteurized milk or blending raw eggs into a protein drink. An estimated nine million individuals choose to drink raw milk each year with low ill effect (estimate by CDC, May 2011). The CDC is a branch of HHS and tied to FDA; why are they on opposite sides of the table on this issue? This is waste and politics at work with numerous health-related issues causing death and disease, waiting for FDA's attention. What is the real problem (milk lobby)? My wife's family in Veracruz, Mexico, sells and provides unpasteurized milk to the locals; and these folks do not get sick or die (they flourish). I do not condone risky behavior; however, this is America, and we can choose to live on the edge for freedom of choice. How about making the consumer sign an acknowledgement of being informed about the possible dangers and letting them choose? The possible danger associated with consuming milk that is unpasteurized depends on the age of the consumer. Vulnerable populations are susceptible to bacteria and viruses found in unpasteurized milk. How do we know these individuals purchasing the bad milk are not heating or cooking this milk before consuming it? The market sells many raw foods meant for cooking, and there are many ways to get food regulation compliance; let's keep it simple, Sam (Keep It Simple Sam).

The Texas State Health Department has an alert level for eating raw Gulf of Mexico oysters and, literally, has a death threshold before a statewide alert is issued (for disease outbreak in oysters and shellfish). I have eaten at taco stands on the streets of Mexico; street-vendor *matambres* from Argentina; live conchas (clam-like bivalve) from a freshwater lake in San Salvador; Brazilian sidewalk barbecue (*churrasco* style); and blood sausage in Germany but lived to tell about it.

Some Central American countries hang their chicken unrefrigerated in open-air markets, and the people survive and thrive in unsafe food-handling conditions. Yes, let's help educate and set higher health standards, but the nanny-state micromanaging style is not exactly working to date, and it's expensive (for government and the market). There is a world of issues to attend to; let's get the most-hazardous conditions facing our nation, like toxins in imported foods and robust bacteriological testing for imported foods. As fresh, potable/drinkable water sources dwindle globally, farmers desperate to water their fields will turn to gray water from poorly treated urban sewage sources.

Bacterial infections are a concern for the United States too. In May 2011, an outbreak of European enterohemorrhagic bacteria, *E. coli* (EHEC), with multiple other bacterial strains and variant outbreak with Shiga-toxin-producing *E. coli* O104 (or STEC O104) occurred. The United States had domestic cases of this come into the country through travelers from abroad. These outbreaks showcase the need for more import vigilance with continued proactive, sensible, sound, science-based domestic-food inspection approaches. Seafood is what I was mainly exposed to in Houston. We had many seafood warehouses, shrimp processors, and bulk frozen food warehouses to inspect on the Gulf of Mexico coastal area. Seafood, if handled incorrectly, can be lethal to humans. One example is histamine formation in Blue fin/yellow fin tuna species. Temperature tags or data loggers are routinely placed on thousand-dollar tuna fillets from Japan to be used for sushi and sashimi in US restaurants. If any tuna species fillet meat is left for too long out of near-freezing temperatures, it forms histamine toxins that are lethal to anyone who eats it. These toxins are not destroyed by heat, so cooking the toxic fish will only make your meal taste good before you are treated for histamine shock and throat-closing agony. Texas has had recent problems with Gulf of Mexico red snapper due to ciguatera fish poison (CFP), which has lasting neurological effects and toxic to all humans. There is nothing better than a snapper Veracruz for dinner; however, I make sure it's a pacific snapper, and now well, I am not sure. The new Food Safety and Modernization Act (FSMA) laws heavily enforce and emphasize seafood safety measures and HACCP concepts. This is truly a global effort with FDA investigators going to the four corners of the globe to inspect food producers.

Passing rates for Seafood HACCP are currently below average at approximately 40 percent (2010). The not-so-funny thing about the Seafood HACCP class is it's based on a book from 2001 that is at best described as vague (industry description). The 2001 HACCP guide allows for subjective interpretation, in my opinion, and many in the industry struggle with the Seafood HACCP regulations. Do a search on Seafood HACCP warning letters and 483 HACCP observations and you will have hundreds to choose from. The FDA has a new fourth-edition HACCP guide that is easier to follow and more industry friendly (Federal Register Notice of Availability on April, 28, 2011). It had not yet been released when I left the agency in March 2011.

The FDA Seafood Division changed a few words around and made more charts and graphs for industry. They are still training the investigators on the old guide (third edition) until the training regimen is updated. If FDA inspectors do not fully understand the HACCP guide and training, how is the seafood industry supposed to grasp the HACCP concept? Congressional mandates for domestic and international food inspections began in 2006. I have hoped that FDA will send out the great public-affairs specialists to inform the public how FDA wants to help make the United States healthy and health conscious.

I parted ways with HACCP inspections in 2003 and focused on BIMO. The district already had an official "BIMO" specialist, but Houston was home to multiple universities involved in Research, so someone local was needed to keep up with the inspection demand. Having another (unofficially recognized) BIMO specialist in the district did not sit well with management, so maybe it is better to be a jack of all trades, master of none. I estimate there are close to seventy or eighty thousand ongoing human clinical trials in the Houston, Texas, area. I know because I reviewed most of the institutional review boards (IRBs) for Houston. The biggest two IRBs in Houston have anywhere from four to six thousand clinical trials under their review. The FDA had at most four investigators, covering BIMO in Houston. The clinical trial to FDA investigator ratio is very high considering that two of the four Houston FDA investigators may get twenty BIMO audits in a year and the rest of the twenty inspections combined with all program areas (food, drugs, device, and biologics). I will be generous and say that the Houston area gets seventy BIMO audits completed, and of those a portion are IRBs or nonhuman clinical trial inspections. You can do the math: thirty thousand clinical trials divided by seventy total inspections equals a Clinical Investigator's odds of getting an FDA inspection in Houston in any given year.

CHAPTER 3

BIMO Training

WHAT DOES BIMO mean and why is it so important, or better yet, what makes me think you or I can review it? Bioresearch monitoring is many reviews all in one acronym. BIMO is the review of Clinical Investigators (medical doctors conducting clinical trials); institutional review boards (IRBs); sponsors (biologic, device, drug maker/innovator); monitors (quality assurance for drug trial); good laboratory practice (GLP, clinical and nonclinical); and bioequivalence and bioavailability clinics/laboratories. BIMO covers all unapproved drugs, devices, and biologics (plus hybrid therapies).

Usually, FDA starts new personnel out in foods and keeps them there a few years. I started out just like everyone else, but very early on I took a slightly different path because my new supervisor and the Dallas District Bioresearch Monitoring (BIMO) specialist recognized my potential to conduct BIMO audits. I took BIMO training in New Orleans (March 1999, around St. Patrick's Day), bright eyed and ready to conduct my first solo BIMO audit. I had so much to learn, and looking back now, I see I was not even ready. At the time, our Houston resident post had two investigators that conducted BIMO audits. One of the investigators (my mentor, Red) was on her way out the door after nine years of dedicated service (she also helped edit this manuscript). I was the only BIMO candidate from my new hire crew at the time. Houston had approximately twenty thousand ongoing human clinical trials (in 2000) in the medical center, and on average, each investigator gets to twenty-two audits a year average (very generous average). I had my BIMO class before basic law and evidence and started going out on BIMO team investigations in April 1999. I admit it was early; but my education, industry experience, and my drive to learn kept me going and not guessing.

The FDA got a deal with me, bringing me in as a GS-5 with a master's in biotechnology and two years' device/drug manufacturing experience. My dad said, "If you do not take this job, you will regret it for the rest of your life"; and he would have been right, the old pharmacist/navy veteran. The emphasis is on domestic self-compliance and international inspection priority. In plain language, the FDA is saying to the US clinical trial industry, "We trust you and will verify only a fraction of your highest-enrolled sites and 30 percent of the subjects' data" (100 percent consent review). I will tell you that I and the Dallas District specialist routinely reviewed all study subject records (adverse events) and all primary and secondary efficacy end points (plus test article review).

If I had a dollar for every time I explained what I do for a living, I would already be rich. BIMO inspections (and now audits) are highly scientific and complex work that demands brainpower and detail orientation. You have got to reverse-engineer every test article in your mind and be able to find that needle in a haystack. In my opinion, each drug, device, or biologic human clinical trial should be monitored and checked by an independent third party (non-study personnel) and then the FDA should conduct the review. Normally, FDA reviews a test article protocol because the application for approval was submitted, the Principal Investigator was pulled off the study, there was a customer injury complaint, or FDA decided to conduct a real-time audit. I cannot tell you how many times I showed up for a device real-time audit and the study was closed or all subjects were completed (they were waiting for data lock). Most FDA investigators do not show the official assignment sheet and claim the audit was routine surveillance. Neither I nor the FDA wants to look funny by stating I am here to conduct a real-time audit on your closed-out clinical trial.

The FDA has an inspection compliance program guidance manual (CPGM) for each type of BIMO audit. All of these CPGMs for BIMO are available on the internet and are numbered as follows: CPGM 7348.811, Clinical Investigator and Sponsor Investigators; CPGM 7348.810, Sponsors and Monitors; CPGM 7348.808, Good Laboratory Practice; CPGM 7348.001 Bioequivalence; and CPGM 7348.809Institutional Review Boards. Here is the BIMO web link for public access to all the CPGMs: *http://www.fda.gov/ScienceResearch/SpecialTopics/ RunningClinicalTrials/ucm160670.htm.*

It's ironic, but if the BIMO centers were a drug or device firm FDA audited, they would get 483 citations for not updating and reviewing internal standard operating procedures for ten years. The Health and Human Service Office of Inspector General

(OIG) feels the same way. The latest or most recent report, to my knowledge, was from an OIG audit conducted on the FDA BIMO program in 2006 and the findings published in 2007 (*http://oig.hhs.gov/oei/reports/oei-01-06-00160.pdf*). Needless to say, FDA did not get a favorable report from the IOG (please read), and many deficiencies were noted. The BIMO process and procedures have not changed much since their inception, and if the FDA implemented OIG corrective actions, the FDA investigators were not provided with documentation or training. FDA has many internal issues to deal with along with the obvious external regulatory job. I was shocked the first time I read the IOG report. I asked myself, how could the HHS OIG give the FDA such an unfavorable report? The FDA simply does not review enough clinical trials real time or have enough trained BIMO staff to cover more than 1 percent of the clinical trials being conducted. The obvious fix is to train more new FDA investigators to conduct BIMO. The downside is that FDA procured the new hires for food work (Congress mandate). Since FDA recently received enhanced food authority, it will flex the newly granted regulatory muscles and set some food precedents. The next step will hopefully be congressionally approved enhanced biologics, device, and drug regulatory authority.

BIMO inspections are NOT easy. I have personally taken many new and seasoned investigators into the field for their first BIMO inspections, and many decided early on that maybe they will only do IRB audits or GLP audits. Some of the investigators decided early in their career that they never want to see another BIMO assignment. We are all different and have different aptitudes for certain program areas and subject matter. I commend anyone who does their job well and with public safety in mind. BIMO is a very specialized program area not for the faint of heart. As a BIMO investigator, you will see patient records, X-rays, MRIs, pictures, surgery reports, and death reports. I cannot tell you how many times I felt despair at the number of human deaths I have seen on paper. Those records were tied to someone's family member or loved one. The FDA did not teach me how to respectfully review patient records, and I took it upon myself to be objective and dignified. The FDA BIMO training teaches individuals to make sure the Clinical Investigator follows the Code of Federal Regulation (CFR) and to evaluate the site per CPGM. I did not receive training on how to deal with death or what the clinician (doctor or research nurse) feels for their patient that did make it through the clinical trial. This is one part of the job FDA needs to train investigators for. In twelve years of conducting BIMO, I have seen possibly more patient records than some doctors have, let's say, in a small-town clinic. You are expected to maintain professional decorum and move to the next project, but human nature pulls you into the patient perspective.

We all, at some point, will be a patient; and hopefully, the attending clinician will not be in a hurry or try to rush you to make a split-second, life-and-death decision. I firmly believe a clinical perspective of compassion and advocacy for the patient should be part of the BIMO training. As I went through many personal family losses from 2001 to 2009, I learned how to struggle with the fact that we have a very short time here on earth. We should try to make a positive footprint and live to our fullest potential.

The FDA now also has a role in regulation of nicotine-containing/tobacco products; HHS will structure health care into the budget and FDA's role in that if any. I wonder why the overlap with the Alcohol, Tobacco, and Firearms (ATF), but that is for Congress to explain. The waste and conglomeration of resources are apparent and must be reviewed by the Government Accounting Office. The Health and Human Services responsibilities have bloated into a megalith with insufficient funds. The focus should be on safe drugs, devices, biologics, and accomplishing BIMOs; but that is just my humble opinion. Many changes lie ahead, and modernization must continue. FDA needs to update many procedures (CPGMs), such as radionuclide medication, electronic records guidance for all regulated industry, bioequivalence, IRBs, and GLP inspection guides.

FDA needs to give much more guidance on hybrid therapeutic devices (drugs, biologics, or device combination products); cell and gene therapy; and nanotechnology applications. The call for e-records submissions from industry should prompt FDA to further clarify and update 21 CFR Part 11 guidance. An FDA report is required after every inspection, and mine are available to you through the Freedom of Information Act (FOIA). Some of the warning letters that I have on file are available on the Internet.

Training for Each BIMO Program Area

BIMO training takes years to complete, and job experience is the main training. There is FDA training for each type of BIMO investigation, and you have to be trained and evaluated before the BIMO program monitor lets you conduct a solo BIMO investigation. During the BIMO training, they usually bring up how to meet and greet your customers and treat the doctors and clinicians with a professional tone. I will admit, when dealing with an MD, PharmD, director of giant hospital system, you may feel out of your league, especially when the hospital lawyers are right in the room to assist and record the inspection. We all have a job to do, and global health is a cooperative effort. Most doctors acknowledge the need for FDA because they only have to look at health-care issues in other countries that do not have robust health oversight.

CPGM 7348.811 Clinical Investigators' training is usually the first program area investigators start with. Houston has more than forty thousand ongoing clinical trials in the medical center and surrounding Houston metro area (2010-2011). The need for Clinical Investigator/Principal Investigator FDA compliance review is high. As an FDA investigator, I averaged twenty-five BIMO audits per year with approximately 90 percent of these inspections as Clinical Investigator for data validation. There were two of us covering the Houston-area BIMOs for all program areas, so I hope this puts the need for BIMO inspections from FDA into perspective for you. In the basic BIMO training course, you get a good overview of each type of inspection with the focus on clinical-investigator-data validation. You are presented with case studies (good and bad inspections), industry deficiency trends, and warning-letter presentations.

The hardest parts of the training are the mock inspection and 483 writing exercises. You get one week to learn how to conduct BIMO inspections. New investigators go through many team inspections (for proficiency evaluation) during the training period. At first, it does not seem possible to let a newbie lose in the world of pharmaceuticals; however, data validation can be done by anyone. If I can be trained to do this job, anyone can do it; ask any of my college classmates or friends. I am not a genius or mega mind. I am highly trained and skilled at what I do, but that has taken twelve years to accomplish.

What is data validation? In essence, the Review Division is conducting the audit through data validation fieldwork and medical review team perspective. Usually, these inspections are prompted by the submission of an NDA. As part of the review process for the application, the reviewers create assignments for field investigators to go to the sites and review data. As an investigator, you get the CPGM as the playbook, the assignment information, and the sponsor data listings. The Review Division is conducting the audit through data validation fieldwork and medical review team perspective. The field investigator is responsible in part for ensuring Clinical Investigators are reporting serious adverse events per time frames, the source data (electronic, clinic evaluations, end point efficacy, and protocol required test results) matches sponsor-provided data listings, and verifying test article accountability. Seasoned BIMO investigators and specialists will review all study subjects and ensure complete regulatory compliance. The on-the-job training teaches field investigators how to review the monitor and deviation correspondence to locate discussion items and 483 observations. Trust, but verify, and regulatory discretion usually apply. In some cases, the deviations are administrative in nature or patient-incurred time frame issues that warrant a discussion item noted in the official report and documentation exhibits from the study correspondence.

I hope and expect more training and certification for the very important BIMO program area. As the centers settle into their new White Oak office building, maybe they will communicate and implement expectations for training new BIMO investigators.

Most of the inspections FDA conducts are clinical-investigator-data validations because those are where the bulk of the work is. I recall many Clinical Investigators looking at me like I was from Mars and asking themselves, "How can this fresh-faced kid be inspecting my important work?" The truth is, the inspection process is compartmentalized and regulated through the assigned center with a final peer team review (MDs, PhD's, and PharmD's) for classification. The center determines no action indicated (NAI), voluntary action indicated (VAI), and official action indicated (OAI). The field investigator gathers the exhibits and reports on data validation (paper and e-data) observations. As required by FDA, I always let my customers know that I was not the final determinant of compliance and that the review team would review the exhibits and my report for the final determination. The Review Division looks at all the investigations for an application to give or deny pending approval. As an investigator, you do not have to be equal in knowledge with your customer (Principal Investigator) to conduct a data-validation audit; you just have to be able to read and understand the protocol. The FDA field investigator is not reviewing the medical practice for your clinic team. The field investigator is ensuring patient safety and informed consent, protocol adherence, CFR compliance, and test-article accountability. Regulatory compliance is easier stated than completed. Being able to read a protocol, find unreported serious adverse events, and any other regulatory compliance issue is hard work. I am not stating that this is easy work, because it is the most complicated work you can do where missed mistakes may cost lives down the line. I am saying that if you put your mind to it and this is your field of choice, you can do this job.

The point I am trying to make is, FDA trains you what to look for and how to look for it with BIMO inspections. The drug and device schools are more intense, and you have to certify in different aspects of those program areas. The BIMO program has not started this phase of certification. The focus is on getting inspections done before user fee act time frames. FDA has been increasing international BIMO inspections for years now. The notion of domestic self-compliance is misguided in the sense that FDA issues many BIMO warning letters each year. I think relying on an enhanced multilevel cooperative between institutional review boards; monitors/ CROs; and the ICH model of mandatory third-party review would solidify a global team effort. FDA should conduct many more BIMO clinical-investigator inspections per year and may be able to achieve this goal if it is a goal. With the FDA mandate of all electronic submissions, your firms will have to migrate to all electronic records. It is possible for an FDA investigator to review the electronic records from their office.

FDA investigators can spot most regulatory issues from the FDA field office, and if a trip to the site is needed in the beginning and end, so be it. I cannot tell you how many times a clinical-investigator site provided me with web access or a CD data. FDA investigators are not allowed to touch a firm's hardware interface. In plain language, we cannot and should not touch your computer terminal. I have been told many times that staff is not available for me to work the computer terminal, at which point I would make a request to speak with the IT team. The IT team would then provide a temporary password for web access or a CD was provided. We do think outside the box and get the job done professionally and, hopefully, politely. You may only see an FDA investigator once in your career, or you may see them every year. I tell you about these electronic records issues because it proves my point on off-site FDA review. I also want to point out the need for FDA to provide better computer-system training to field investigators and regulated industry.

CPGM 7348.810 covers Sponsors and Monitors including contract research organizations (CROs). CROs are currently in FDA's crosshairs and have been for over two years. CROs with less-than-adequate staff and facilities to conduct human clinical trials are receiving warning letters and other regulatory penalties. The FDA has not conducted a good sponsor or CRO inspection blitz in many years. I have routinely seen study sites get warning letters because monitors did not catch informed consent violations early in the trial or for regulatory and subject record-keeping violations. Catching serious problems early in the trial will prevent adverse events and save time and money in the long run. You do not want to throw study data out due to errors and inconsistent data. Your return on investment will always be high if regulatory compliance is built in to your projects and systems.

I have observed CROs collecting original-source site documentation from the clinic site at study closeout. I wonder how CROs miss the basic reason FDA investigators conduct data-validation audits! FDA wants to validate that all original source documentation match the case report form (CRF) and the sponsor-provided data listing, efficacy end points, and adverse-event lists. CROs can easily scan the original source documents into their system, but physically removing the source documents has conditions. If a CRO truly wants the original documents for whatever reason, the CRO may certify each copy as a true duplicate of the original (21 CFR describes this process). In many cases, the Clinical Investigator relocates, or there is no available space and money to store the records, so the sponsor may step in to take over. As long as the FDA can follow the paper trail and review original documents, there is no problem.

Copies may and have been found to be falsified, so investigators will usually not review paper copies of paper source records. Electronic printout (output) is a different way to operate now and is acceptable for review.

The FDA did not expend very much time training us to conduct sponsor or monitor audits because in early 2000, the FDA did not conduct very many of these type of audits. The FDA is now beginning to understand that protocol violations and deviations have a direct correlation to the amount of oversight a clinical trial has. FDA may now be training the newer investigators on more case studies and 483 trends for sponsor and monitor audits. Most of my experience has been on-the-job training by conducting the inspections based on the compliance program and specific assignment requests. The Dallas District, in general, does not have many sponsors in the geographic area, but does have many CRO companies big and small. I inspected many CROs during my time at FDA. During the last few years, FDA has ramped up CRO inspections to ensure qualified individuals are doing the monitoring work at clinic sites (2010-2011). The FDA also wants to make sure Principal Investigators (PI) are not delegating medical procedures (MD only) to non-medical, or otherwise non-qualified personnel.

I have seen too many PIs delegating medical observation work to research nurses or CROs with English majors. In many cases, the sponsor will qualify CROs before the PI can delegate any study procedures. I can tell you that FDA audits any complaint or subject injury connected to sponsors or monitors, which used to comprise the bulk of audits on these firms. The FDA has started a blitz on inspections for sponsors and monitors that will only be ramped up. If you build quality into your systems from start to finish, you should get a quality product result. This means if sponsors and monitors are implementing quality systems and have qualified medically trained staff, projects will at least start with quality. All of you sponsors and monitors get ready for your FDA audits because this is current news for you. CROs, the FDA will ensure that your projects are being adequately reviewed and your operation is compliant. FDA will audit your study data validation, annual/progress reporting, test-article labeling, and manufacturing processes, if not contracted out. Your most significant risk/vulnerable-population test articles will be selected every time. Major change is on the horizon, and the sleeping giant is waking up to regulate.

CPGM 7348.808 regards Good Laboratory Practice (GLP), Nonclinical. This program area is vital to drug development and discovery. FDA provides the investigator with a week of training in a real lab setting with hands-on review of equipment, animal care and necropsy, records maintenance, and test-article accountability. The FDA offers the seasoned BIMO investigators with advanced GLP nonclinical, which was updated. The FDA clearly understands that these are the test article's proving grounds and help to establish toxicity profiles. FDA typically inspects GLP operations once every two years. It seems many GLP firms are taking on more EPA-regulated studies to supplement business. GLP firms were more than happy to show me their EPA side of operations. I observed many aquatic studies, freshwater and saltwater, due to Houston's proximity to the Gulf Coast. I really enjoyed not having to wear a suit and tie in Houston for GLP inspections. The assignment usually requested three or four GLP studies for review, and I would review six or seven if they had that many. To me, GLP is by nature an important part of the process because this is where the test article is given a profile and possible adverse-event listings (drugs and biologics). Device GLP significant-risk test articles for in vivo implantable devices must go through biocompatibility and safety studies (tissue interaction). Clinical in-vitro diagnostics get a pass on this part of the process. Very few districts have device-biocompatibility laboratories to inspect. This type of inspection is done more internationally and, as with other industries, has gone east. Most inspections are conducted on chemical and biological test articles. Most of my experience is with pharmaceutical test articles (with numbers and name designations). Toxicity studies and adverse-event discovery conducted under GLP compliance are the cornerstones to finding safe and effective test articles for the market.

GLP is recognizably important to FDA, and updated and enhanced GLP-compliance field guidance (last issued 2001 to date) is long overdue. Industry may want to be proactive and start this discussion to get the FDA guidance ball rolling. The main issue is that many centers have a say in GLP, and everyone is very "busy." FDA centers, let's get to work and hammer this out because more than a decade has passed us by. When you are in FDA, you do not have a forum to speak with all the centers about these types of issues. Let's be honest; would the centers really want to hear anything from the frontline grunt in the field? (Ask an army general this question.) The open forum is a transparent dialogue that has to be a two-way discussion. Transparency written in procedures but lacking in substance or implementation is just more empty hot air.

I am not an expert; however, I have been trained to review procedures and processes, FDA's included.

CPGM 7348.809, covers Institutional Review Boards (IRBs.) The FDA, Department of Health and Humans Services Office for Human Research Protections (OHRP), and many other Government Accounting Office agencies (GAO) are looking to enhance IRB oversight. FDA typically assigns the IRB work through one of the centers, and around six or seven ongoing clinical trials are reviewed. The compliance program calls for three studies to be reviewed at minimum. If the IRB audit turns regulatory, the sky is the limit. The investigator may be there for weeks, reviewing ten or twenty approved protocols. This is still a fraction of the work most IRBs do. Most IRBs typically have hundreds or thousands of approved clinical trials under their review. One might ask how the FDA even finds anything wrong with IRBs? The FDA trains investigators to track and trend IRB trouble spots by reviewing the most-vulnerable population and highest-risk clinical trials. You may be asking yourself, are six or seven studies enough for a robust review? I asked myself that same question, and in most cases, it will be sufficient. The compliance program requires that for those studies reviewed at an IRB, you look at everything. What is everything? Everything is the approved protocol versions, test-article description, meeting minutes for all approvals, discussion points, safety data updates, serious adverse-event reporting (per protocol), informed consents, annual reports, protocol-violation reports, regulatory documents, and study-closure documentation. This is not an all-inclusive list, and you may refer to the compliance program for the full description.

I will tell you that when you go to an IRB and ask for this documentation, it may fill the room you are in. It will seem like too much to do in a week's time. FDA does not currently inspect foreign/international IRBs because their regulatory basis and requirements are not the same as those in the US. The FDA updated the Compliance Program in late 2011. I will repeat this feeling of "FDA's job is too important globally, it cannot fail." IRBs should feel like part of the QA team instead of the next interrogation subject.

All the centers should get together and work on some talking points and break up the IRB CPGM into program areas with intense focus areas of trended data that is current. The field investigators' review for IRBs should be up to eight or nine protocols reviewed with each program area included in the audit with emphasis on vulnerable-population human clinical trials. Special emphasis should be given to central IRB review for complete compliance with 21 CFR regulations. Central IRBs should have a community member from each of the clinical trials under review and be conducting on-site QA reviews to ensure regulatory compliance. Large institutional IRBs should be reviewed annually to cover more of the thousands of studies they review with FDA-IRB team-development emphasis. As IRB protocol-review inventory goes up, so should the amount of FDA oversight. The amount of human clinical trials increases, and so does the gap in QA coverage from FDA and IRBs. As a team, you can control, track, and trend to win. As two separate teams, you struggle to keep cost down for new hires and work the employees you have triple, with employee overturn as the outcome.

CPGM 7348.001 regards Bioequivalence. During the weeklong BIMO basic training, very little time is spent on the bioequivalence program. The FDA should develop and enhance field-investigator training in this area of BIMO. If the field investigator does not have mass spectrometry LC/MS/MS training, then there is much to learn before your first inspection. The field investigator does not usually conduct bioequivalence inspections alone for this very reason. A center expert (Pharm D, PhD, or MD) usually reviews all the technical data and validation aspects of the inspection. Field investigators would be able to accomplish some of the technical review if they were trained. I was able to assist in the technical review for many inspections due to mass spectrometry exposure in graduate studies and my work as an incoming raw-materials technician in the drug field. If FDA did provide more training for field investigators in the bioequivalence program, more studies could be reviewed at one time, and more firm inspections could be accomplished. The field investigator is the lead but mainly reviews laboratory equipment compliance, subject, collection reports (CRs), sample review, and employee training records.

That more training is needed with regard to the BIMO program is an understatement. I consistently requested nanotech and biotechnology training, which was always in Washington DC. I was denied every request due to lack of funds. It is not easy to persuade upper district management that you need this type of training. The focus should be on getting the work done and training on future technology already in the pipeline. How much work is really getting done by FDA? I want you to search for the answer to that question.

I challenge you to do some research, fact-find, and seek transparency. My FDA training record is provided for you at the end of this book. The current FDA way of "Learn as you go" may not be the best way to train the new crew. Mentoring is a vital part of new hire training, and FDA is trying to implement a nationwide mentor program for new hires. We could spend much more time here in the training area because we all need more training balanced into our work-program area.

One major stumbling block for FDA training is that most FDA trainers are FDA national experts or district specialist field-workers. These individuals are stretched to the limit with international FDA work, district work, and training internal and private industry. You have to add the whole equation for the trainers because they are traveling approximately 40 percent and need time off. Life happens for them and their families, so schedules get tight with no flexibility. I have observed more third-party trainers used lately for highly technical aspects of FDA training.

This is a positive trend, but FDA likes to keep a handle on every aspect of training so that no lines are crossed. Many of the third-party trainers are ex-FDA so that all parties know what is expected, and test cases are kept confidential in public trust. FDA trainers like to use old inspections that may have been flawed or good inspections that went to regulatory status as examples of final work product. Many times the names are removed from work product so there is no embarrassment. FDA has a very small feel and family-like atmosphere. I have heard the center is a rugged operating terrain but never made it to the White Oak Crystal Palace. I have suggested to upper management many times that FDA should send field investigators to the center to work there in a light rotation-style review effort. FDA does not train investigators on specific human body systems or therapy types. FDA trains you to validate data and find discrepancies. As a BIMO investigator you see any and all therapy types in many different phases of the application process. Updating procedures and training BIMO investigators will be an issue for the foreseeable future. The FDA management and employee unions constantly try to balance the training needs of both new hires and seasoned field investigators. Management should understand that it would not take away from field investigators' FDA ORA work. There is too much work for current FDA field BIMO staff plus enough for an army of contract BIMO reviewers.

The FDA will still have the final say on test-article approval and can easily audit QA contractors. If the approximate amount of 15 percent approval rate for test articles is accurate, why not review 30 percent for good coverage? This can be done by throwing out prehistoric notions of status quo and getting to work. There are too many skeptics out there; let's reinvent the wheel and protect the public. I understand the need for oversight and providing a quality work product, but not if it slows down an already-slow system. Pick up the snail pace and get the troops out into the field. We all have a gift to share, and I will talk about this more in the last chapter. You cannot be good at all things, FDA, because FDA regulates a world of goods and services.

Most FDA investigators try to accomplish mastery of two program areas. As a newbie, you get to choose what program areas you would like to work in. As time goes on, the investigator is trained and observed for aptitude in the program areas of choice. I stayed in the BIMO area in order to gain as much aptitude and experience during my time at FDA. At every step, I was second-guessed many times and handpicked to do other work. In the end, there were too many BIMOs to conduct in Houston and someone had to complete it on time. Management likes to get you out of your comfort zone so you can do more with less. I got so tired of the get-out-of-your-comfort-zone speech. It is not comfortable to conduct FDA business, and they want to dilute what you do best. I say we all have a talent and management should exploit what the individual is good at because it's logical. Let's continue down the yellow brick highway.

CHAPTER 4

BIMO Inspections

FDA BIMO INVESTIGATORS are asked to conduct data validation, for-cause clinical-investigator inspections, IRB records and study review, GLP nonclinical inspections, sponsor and monitor specific or random inspections, and bioequivalence inspections. If that sounds like a lot of work, you're wrong; it is a BOATLOAD of work. Each BIMO program area has a specific plan of action and FDA trends 483 observations, so investigators have focused review areas for each type of inspection. FDA has released to the public websites detailing regulatory trends: *http://www.fda.gov/iceci/EnforcementActions/ucm250720.htm*.

The FDA is also stating a commitment to transparency in the following public domain website: *http://www.fda.gov/AboutFDA/Transparency/default.htm*

Clinical-investigator audits are the bulk of my BIMO experience and the domestic focus area for the BIMO program area. FDA is painfully aware the BIMO inspection program is tied to user fee money that fuels the rising operating costs. Congress is currently mandating more food inspections. I have not quite figured out how the Department of Agriculture gets a pass on the food workload, but Congress runs the show. FDA Investigators are now mandated to complete some food-program work regardless of their specialty. The BIMO work will decrease in number under the current congressional food mandate. A good balance among all program areas is a challenging endeavor that should not be determined by politics, in my opinion. At a time when more BIMO inspections are needed, less will be conducted. In industry, quality assurance is separated from operations. Congress mandating more food work from one agency is counterproductive toward the other program areas FDA needs to focus on. More than one agency overlaps with FDA on inspecting food production, and the cooperative effort should be enhanced. One agency should not be burdened with the heavy lifting when it is already asked to do more program areas than it can handle with the current staff level. There have always been rumors about FDA splitting into two separate organizations, foods and drugs. I am not so sure this idea would work. I do know that when you have ten-year-old BIMO procedures to operate from, more focus is needed on that area. The FDA will always be underfunded and undermanned, but it is what they do with those funds and assets that will determine success in accomplishing the mission. FDA moves forward cautiously and deliberately with focus on public safety and industry comment. I would not suggest speeding the process up or down because this clinical science-based approach is deliberate with proven safety results.

BIMO inspections are generated by the health-therapeutics centers, and I was happy to deal directly with the centers. The district program areas (biologics, food, drugs, and devices) travel an uphill, sometimes political, battle for regulatory action. District politics and second-guessing can stopgap good cases from seeing the light of day. The district Compliance Division in general is a reactionary force in nature. When a "hot" case with regulatory observations that warrants FDA action gets handed to Compliance, they take over. The "hot" case is then developed, and the center legal department does a review to ensure FDA has a presentable case for the federal court system. A current book about the FDA Office of Enforcement Compliance Division national and district case development should be written. I did not get a chance to interact with Dallas District Compliance during my career, so I cannot make too many comments here. I did, however, interact with the BIMO center compliance divisions for CBER, CDER, and CDRH during my entire career. Compliance at the district level does the best it can with the few it has on staff. Dallas District has hundreds of field investigators and seven or eight compliance officers, so you can do the math. It is frustrating to say the least when, as an investigator, you find the needle in a haystack and develop a good case only for the needle to get lost in the district Compliance haystack.

FDA district managers have asked us "why doesn't industry take us seriously"? My answer was always because we give the same 483 observations over and over with very few warning letters or tangible legal actions. Maybe if FDA district Compliance developed more actionable cases and provided industry with guidance on how to correct the 483 observations, a more serious tone would follow. I have found that many times, food firms do not understand in plain language what the 483 observation is, or they need some less-legal explanation of the corrective actions. Many times, language gets in the way. Firms that knowingly and willingly produce harmful products for the market, FDA will find you. FDA district Compliance Branch started having meetings and conferences with firms around 2006. Compliance understands that industry wants to comply with FDA to stay in business, and this process yields results. This process does work because dialogue produces guidance for industry. It is very easy to tell someone "You're doing it wrong," and it is very difficult to tell someone how to do the job right without consulting. FDA is not a consulting business, but the FDA consults every day with private industry. FDA field investigators are asked to give guidance without consulting in plain language. Field investigators are not robots, and as humans, we all do things in a different way.

Data validation is a process that takes many pieces of a protocol puzzle to be laid out and put together. The FDA medical reviewers should be specialists in the body system covered so the field investigator does data validation only. I tried to explain force multiplication to the Argentina Health Ministry heads, but I may not have been coherent. They looked at me like, *How is this Tex-Mex-looking kid even doing his job?* A few minutes later, when I spoke to them, it was like *okay, he knows the FDA regulations, but how can we set this program up in our country to effectively approve test articles?* It seems that most countries try to employ medically trained professionals (physician assistant, nurse, doctor, or pharmacologist), which might be ideal. I am a proof that you can conduct data validation and medical review to get the job done. I say, yes, employ the medically trained professionals to oversee dozens of scientifically minded data-validation specialists. I will say again, a graduate degree in biochemistry or life science and higher will speed up the training process. I would estimate that it took me four years to become proficient at BIMO program investigations and six years to achieve program situational awareness. Most of my customers will, hopefully, tell you that I changed their mind about the so-called FDA bullies. Even when the news was bad, I tried to be a goodwill ambassador to every one of the professionals I worked with. I will continue to treat my customers with respect and goodwill because we have a big job to do.

Data validation is no small talking point; it is the difficult task of reevaluating source documentation (all of it) with nice, neat data listings and biostatistical endpoints. I tried to read each protocol at least three times in order to start a clinical-investigator inspection. I routinely did Internet and FDA library searches on biologics, devices, and drugs because if you do not understand the test article, you cannot conduct a complete BIMO audit. I know BIMO program specialists are needed when so many firms in 2011 asked me what is considered source documentation during an official inspection (before I left). It is the most basic principle of any scientific experiment to document every aspect of the process. Source is typically considered the first location that a data point is recorded. If for some reason your staff writes a subject's vital signs on a napkin, that napkin is now considered source documentation. If your staff takes the information and inputs that data into a computer, the napkin is still considered source. If your staff discards the napkin, your clinical site just destroyed source documents. When FDA does go to your firm for an investigation, they will find out your process. If the FDA investigator observes that your system was to write the vitals on a napkin then input the data; you will likely have to present the napkin in the source documents or receive a 483 observation. Clinical sites must retain any and all sources of clinical-trial documentation in all formats for FDA inspection as required by your 1572 statement, or investigator contract.

I would invariably go straight for any major violations within the first day of inspection, leaving the rest of the time for discussion and evidence development. Experience has trained me well, and I hope to continue test-article QA for your products. I continue to learn about new and emerging health products and wait for the FDA to update BIMO.

Principal Investigator inspections from FDA must increase for two reasons: (1) user fee monies are used to fund FDA and much more funding is needed, and (2) human clinical trials are increasing exponentially in number worldwide – not decreasing. FDA traditionally has been reactionary in nature with waves of real-time inspection blitz initiatives per center. I have often wondered why I was conducting inspections on information that was locked and closed out two or three years ago. If violations occur that affect the end point efficacy data, it is too late to correct them or retroactively amend any data. The whole study has to be redone or just thrown out. It almost seems counterproductive but more like sink or swim for industry. FDA typically inspects a Clinical Investigator one time for application approvals, so if they go in for phase 1 review, the trial site will not be looked at again in phase 3 unless there is a complaint or the PI is disqualified for compliance. Limited manpower will always be a factor with regard to the amount of inspections that get completed or assigned. Most Clinical Investigators may only get inspected once or twice in their long careers, and some get reviewed every other year.

I have had many first-time inspections where the PI stated, "I never thought I would see an FDA investigator in my clinic." I always explained they had nothing to get stressed about and that I would be done as quickly as possible (quick and painless). I tried to be like the good nurse that vaccinates you so fast there is nothing to cry about. I stressed that the PI should attend to the patients first and, if I had questions for the end of the day, to stop by as time permitted. The patients always come first, and my FDA questions or concerns may be addressed accordingly. Most of the time, I was able to answer the questions through review of records and only had questions when observations were encountered. I always presented my findings early in the inspections in order to give the clinic team time for a response or acknowledgment and corrective-action plan.

With the advent of all electronic records, FDA can perform early electronic-records review and a late-stage on-site inspection with current resources and staff. Clinical-research sites many times are understaffed and do not have time to sit with FDA investigators. It is very difficult to conduct an all-electronic review when you are not allowed to operate the clinical-site terminal. The result will be either a DVD or a web-link-access review.

I want to mention and thank the many professional and overworked research-coordinator clinical staff I have inspected. The research coordinators and clinic staff do the heavy lifting at many human clinical-research sites. The personalized medicine clinics have more PI and sub investigator data-entry participation due to limited staff or by choice. I did see some PIs that wanted to be involved in every aspect of the clinical trial. However, those PIs were not professors at the medical school conducting four and five research trials and running two or three clinics. You, ladies and gentlemen, are machines; but seriously, take some time off. Rest, relax, and heal your mind and body. You are human like us all. I have observed and interviewed many research coordinators that were conducting more than five ongoing clinical trials without much support staff. The 21 CFR does not micromanage study sites; but common sense and logic should dictate that clinic staff need to eat, sleep, and have time off. We are not robots! Once again, I will say you need sleep, whether you want it or not. If your clinic has high turnover and low morale (equals low productivity), you either lower your ongoing trials or bring up the staff levels (maybe mandate vacation). Ensure your projects succeed with highly trained staff with sufficient support to conduct the workload. I may be able to help you with employee retention and vacation incentives.

I focused on three areas during every clinical-investigator FDA review:

My first area of focus was human-subject protection throughout the study period. An important entity of the review is the informed-consent form (ICF), documentation of a process critical in every human clinical trial. The ICF process incorporates in plain, well-defined language the study procedures, possible risks, confidentiality, and voluntary aspect of research (there are seven). Serious adverse-event reporting within protocol time frames is very crucial for subject protection. Experienced, medically trained professionals must perform the initial inclusion and exclusion process of the clinical trial. I have written and issued many 483 observation forms to Principal Investigators for inclusion and exclusion violations (for not following the protocol). This is a patient-safety issue and is taken seriously by the FDA centers. Patients that do not meet the indication for the test article could be at risk for serious adverse event (drug, device or biologic). Many clinics use in-house patients; however, many new clinical trials are requesting naive study subjects with no previous clinical-trial entry. Assuring your study subjects meet inclusion and do not meet exclusion is the most basic aspect of your clinical trial; get it right the first time and every time. Someone like me will find your violations; we always do.

Second, as previously mentioned, protocol adherence is the second focus area during an FDA inspection. I would always look at the research-team signature list to determine how many research coordinators were involved with the study from start to finish. The turnover rate is a quick indicator of any possible training issues or lapse in good oversight.

How much and how well the study was monitored is another indicator of a successful or noncompliant clinic site. Smaller start-up biologics/biotech, device, and drug sponsors may lack assets for regular monitoring visits and rigorous site training. There will always be a direct correlation between the amount and quality of monitoring and the successful outcome of your clinical trial. Study subject compliance with follow-up visits will always be an issue. Study subjects have lives, and life happens to all of us. As an FDA investigator, I would see this issue at almost every study site that had more than a year's worth of study visits. Investigator discretion is allowed for this, and I did not issue too many 483 observation forms for this deviation. I always noted the issues when observed through exhibits or notations in my report.

Vulnerable-population studies with elderly and very young study patients were usually the worst offenders of missed or late visits out of the protocol window. I always used common sense and logic to dictate my actions for these issues. I have two beautiful children that make my life so crazy. It is hard to get these lovable monsters to cooperate with simple requests like, "Let's put on your clothes," or "Let's eat healthy veggies to get energy and fuel." So I understand that let's-go-to-the-doctor visit for my clinical trial may not happen on time. I did always check for certified letters if stated in the protocol or telephone call log for lost to follow-up subjects. The lost to follow-up procedures were also a part of my standard review.

Every protocol is unique with specific end point efficacy and bio statistical variables. The goal of human clinical research is to minimize variables and collect data to indicate whether a test article is safe and effective.

Third, test-article accountability sounds like a job to be delegated to the pharmacy alone, but it is not. Principal Investigators (PI) are ultimately responsible for every test article that comes into their site. I have been to many FDA inspections where the PI did not review the test-article accountability until the end of the trial. The test-article accountability process is an integral ongoing part of clinical trials. In most cases, even with blinded trials, the PI should be knowledgeable and keep track of the test-article accountability. I have observed sponsors providing a blinded accountability number set for the PI to review and keep track of. There are many 21 CFR-compliant ways to maintain the test-article blind and allow the PI to review what comes in, what is dispensed, and what is destroyed or sent back at closeout. This should be detailed in the protocol. I have issued a fair amount of 483 observations pertaining to test-article accountability and record maintenance. As an FDA investigator, I always took appropriate time to review documentation for all incoming test articles (depending on length of study and number of test articles used). This test article review included storage conditions, dispensing, labeling, expiration date, and the number of destroyed or sent back drug/device/ biologic products. It took days to fully review test-article accountability for some complicated/novel therapy or lengthy clinical trials.

FDA mandates that field investigators adequately review and report on test-article accountability as referenced in compliance program CP7348.811 Clinical Investigator and Sponsor investigators. The point for me was not to find and document discrepancies. The point was always patient safety, protocol adherence, and documented test-article accountability. I tried to view each test article as though it may be used on my family members or a friend. I always maintained my professional decorum. Although I tried to focus on the task at hand and put every other thought aside, I constantly had to block out management issues and administrative demands that absorbed too much of my limited time. I just wanted to be in the field, conducting my reviews and writing my turbo electronic field reports. During my last two years with FDA, I had to spend approximately 30 percent of my time doing administrative work and quality management accountability. Internal FDA Dallas district politics and management-glory agendas irritated me. FDA is a science-based health centered organization where politics and personal gain have no place in the global health mission.

During institutional review board (IRBs) audits, I typically reviewed at least six protocols, and I did more than the CPGM or assignment asked for. If an IRB is reviewing and approving over one hundred or twenty thousand human clinical trials, the guide tells investigators to review at least four FDA-regulated clinical trials. It is a good thing the Office for Human Research Protections (OHRP, *http://www.hhs. gov/ohrp*) is now conducting IRB oversight and providing accreditation for IRBs. FDA needs compliant IRB oversight to monitor more clinical trials in its place. The FDA does not expend a lot of training man-hours for IRB audits, and every center has to take a turn at getting its IRB inspections done. I would always review clinical protocols from each available center so they would all get credit and review oversight. I would review high-risk device protocols and vulnerable-population studies. IRBs are a very important part of FDA oversight and a much-needed asset. IRBs are getting more ICH audits and vendor-qualification review, which should help them remain in compliance with FDA. FDA benefits from IRBs in good regulatory standing to review the many studies FDA field investigators will not be able to inspect. This cooperative effort will increase human clinical-research ethics and patient-safety oversight. FDA provides guidance to IRBs, explaining all BIMO program areas, especially significant-risk-device requirements.

The Government Accounting Office (GAO) has been inspecting IRB ethics practices. Here is a link to GAO report GAO-09-448T focusing on some IRB's failing oversight practices and unethical practices. According to the website *http:// www.gao.gov/new.items/d09448t.pdf*, the GAO observed that "IRB oversight is vulnerable to unethical manipulation, which elevates the risk that experimental products are approved for human subject tests without full and appropriate review." No doubt, you have heard the story of Coast IRB? GAO investigators created fictitious companies, used counterfeit documents, and invented a fictitious medical device to investigate three key aspects of the IRB system. This review of Health and Human Service directed protection agencies documents huge gaps in patient safety during clinical trials and the need for enhanced internal government oversight. The HHS failures documented by the GAO and Office of Inspector General audits may result in serious adverse events and patient safety violations going undocumented.

GAO also registered its bogus IRB with HHS, and used this registration to apply for an HHS-approved assurance for GAO's fictitious medical device company. (An assurance is a statement by researchers to HHS that their human subject's research will follow ethical principles and federal regulations, which is required before researchers can receive federal funding for the research.) On its assurance application, GAO designated its bogus IRB as the IRB that would review the research covered by the assurance. Even though the entire process was done online or by fax without any human interaction HHS approved the assurance for GAO's fictitious device company. With an HHS-approved assurance, GAO's device company could have applied for federal funding for human subjects research.

FDA and OHRP will also have to increase regulatory diligence and oversight for IRBs. The Health and Human Services Office of the Inspector General (OIG) internal affairs agents may follow up on the GAO deficiencies at OHRP and FDA. There are many proposed bioresearch monitoring IRB changes that should be implemented, but it may be a few more years until FDA has comprehensive CDRH, CDER, and CBER input. The FDA requirements for enhanced QA and mandated ethics oversight will be inevitable. The FDA needs to increase IRB review and oversight with regard to reviewing all program areas under oversight by the IRB. This enhanced FDA review must reinforce the IRBs team membership with regards to patient safety and protocol compliance. The FDA Center Directors know all too well the amount of clinical trials reviewed by field BIMO investigators/reviewers is unacceptable. The way it works right now at FDA is each center gets a turn assigning IRB audits during a two-year inspection cycle. The center that assigns the inspection may want all of the program hour credits. In plain language, if CDRH assigns the IRB BIMO inspection, all of the clinical trials the FDA Investigator reviews have to be a device protocol. What happens if the IRB you inspect reviews one device trial a year and hundreds of drug or biologic protocols? The simple plan would be to audit every program area, with a review of at least three clinical trials per program area. Every center gets credit each audit cycle and the FDA assures the IRB is compliant with all program area regulations.

The compliance program is very clear with regard to IRB inspections and exhibits requested during an FDA inspection. More work is always required when 483 observations are encountered to ensure defensible legal action is required. FDA field investigators are required to treat every inspection as though it will go to court, and many do. Labeling exhibits collected during an inspection is one of the least-favorite jobs an investigator performs because it is tedious and extremely time-consuming. I would like to know why in 2011 the FDA still requires field investigators to hand-count and physically label each exhibit? Every FDA office has scanners and copy/fax machines, which can automate this process. I have spent countless hours in the past twelve years counting and labeling exhibits I collected during my inspections. I bring this up in this section because any field investigator that has accomplished an IRB BIMO knows that you collect stacks of paper with you as exhibits for the report. Due to this issue, I stopped taking the whole protocol or the whole investigator brochure for no-action-indicated (NAI) inspections. I would collect the first five pages of a large document required for review if no violations were observed. I would rather save trees, tax money, and time when it comes to collecting paper exhibits. The compliance program guidance manual (CPGM) is clear on this aspect of less is better for no-action inspections. I would also encourage my counterparts to relax on the paper with the final resulting work product acceptable to the center and district management.

The FDA is testing an all-electronic report submission. However, "slow" and "stop" are the current progress-documentation buzzwords. I expect a lot from the highly professional organization that is FDA because FDA expects much more from regulated industry. Lead by example, or do not call yourself a leader at all. There should be more science-based decisions as opposed to politically based decisions. FDA is not run like a business; however, a product (inspections) is the result. It is great to debate science and fact-based outcomes. If you mix politics with science, you might as well just go to Vegas (lost wages). My father loves Vegas, and I cannot say I have not had my good times there – for work purposes, of course.

Bioethics and human clinical trials should be current focus areas for all IRBs. The FDA is taking note of which IRBs have strong bioethics discussions and ethics members on its staff. I have asked many IRB administrators and chairpersons about their IRB's ethics discussions and meeting minute notations on clinical trial ethics (during routine inspections). I recall receiving pale, blank responses because there were no ethics personnel on the IRB board. FDA does not require IRBs to have ethicists on staff, but do not be surprised when it is required guidance in the 21 CFR. Many changes are on the way as more government oversight agencies to get involved with bioresearch patient protection. In the EMA regulations, IRBs are called independent ethics committees (IECs). Ethics is a focus area for EMA IRB inspections. The EMA website details for the public their guidance documents for inspecting IRBs/IECs. FDA will more than likely consult with every center involved with review of IRBs and the EMA before making any major changes to the IRB compliance program.

CDRH has the most guidance to add simply because IRBs get more 483s for device-review violations than any other center. I will not specifically go into compassionate-use device or high-risk devices because again I want you to possibly contract me for help. I will say that significant risk is more than often deferred to the sponsor. IRBs do not rely on the sponsors' interpretation of significant risk, and do your own research on the device product your IRB is about to approve for human use. Most IRBs conducting oversight of human-device trials must constantly stay on top of the changes in the device regulations. IRBs conducting device-trial oversight should enhance quality assurance audits and real-time on-site compliance review. There is a world of work to do in the device area for all of us. FDA will be rapidly changing industry guidance for IRBs so be ready to implement enhanced program specific guidance.

Most IRBs have a department or team looking at the informed-consent form (ICF) elements. I would hope that all IRBs in operation are combing each ICF for the required elements and reviewing the process as well. I am not letting you off the hook here, IRBs. You must do more because FDA cannot. Human clinical research is an honorable field to work in; however, it comes with great ethical responsibility.

Do not merely follow the CFR/ICH/GCP guidelines when authorizing clinical trials. Go above and beyond to ensure safety and efficacy – the main goal in human clinical research. The informed-consent process continues from the patient's signature to their completion of the clinical trial. The FDA compliance program requires informed consent form (ICF) review and exhibit collection from every protocol reviewed during an IRB inspection. I cannot over-emphasize how important the ICF process is to human clinical research studies. If an IRB or clinic site does get one of the few consent form 483 observations, their customers and peers will take notice. The FDA goes after ICF core element violations/missing elements with full force. There is NO EXCUSE for one of the required ICF elements to be missing from a human clinical trial ICF. Nobody's perfect, but this is such a basic thing that it is ridiculous to miss it (clinical trials 101).

One of my focus areas during an IRB audit was QA review conducted by qualified IRB or third-party staff. I observed IRBs with a team of QA-only staff and some multitasking staff doing a little bit of everything. I will tell you, the IRBs that did not have a dedicated QA staff received far more 483 observations when I left the building. I cannot stress the importance of having a robust autonomous QA review of at least 10 or 15 percent of your ongoing clinical trials annually. The EMA and ICH guidance documents require third-party QA review for human clinical trials. FDA is leaning more and more toward ICH and global standards. It is the IRB's responsibility to ensure the approved human-research projects are following the 21 CFR. How does an IRB ensure 21 CFR compliance without QA oversight and on-site inspections? There is a very short window of opportunity for me here to suggest proactive change. The FDA will come out with more guidance and regulation for IRBs because it has to. As the test articles and hybrid medical therapies evolve, so must the FDA regulations.

IRBs are charged with completing an enormous workload and are, more often than not, the only ethical and QA review a clinical trial may get, the last gatekeeper on a long, winding road to market. I also think nonclinical good laboratory practices (GLP) study information and related toxicity study data should be part of the IRB review (IRB CPGM). I have observed many IRBs requesting nonclinical GLP and toxicity studies. The FDA does not clearly specify review of the GLP information. The CPGM should also have a section for each center to incorporate specific test-article focus areas. Preclinical studies are not required from the device industry. Some device sponsors do conduct high-risk, in vivo device GLP nonclinical studies. It is not only cost appropriate to conduct nonclinical trials, but also, the human risk factor is mitigated as device failures are observed early. FDA will require tissue-interaction studies for hybrid therapy devices.

Next, Nonclinical Good Laboratory Practice (GLP) inspections are very important for FDA and test-article development. I have seen a disturbing trend in which domestic GLP firms are being bought out or conglomerating, only to be internationally outsourced. The GLP firm pool is shrinking domestically, and human clinical trials are increasing worldwide. This is a contradiction in terms of need and economic growth domestically. Normally, GLP firms get an FDA inspection every three years or less, depending on the project output. I can say for certain that I have conducted around twelve GLP inspections throughout my FDA career, which is the least amount for any of my program areas. Many of the GLP firms I inspected had three times more EPA-regulated studies than FDA-regulated studies. The FDA regulations do not overlap, so field investigators do not review EPA-regulated GLP trials. Many of the GLP firms I inspected were more than happy to show me their EPA GLP operations, and I was happy to learn something new, if time permitted. FDA does a fair job training field investigators to conduct GLP inspections. The Dallas District I worked in had a handful of GLP firms, and now that number is dwindling fast. It will now take the international inspections BIMO team to review more GLP firms. The FDA GLP nonclinical compliance program will be updated to align with stringent ICH and EMA standards. Make sure, domestically and internationally, that your GLP firm is ready for the enhanced shift in FDA inspections.

FDA's inspection focus for GLPs is the quality assurance unit review, personnel training, data validation, animal care, Institutional Animal Care and Use Committee (IACUC), amount of FDA-regulated projects, data validation, and test-article storage. Electronic records and paper-record storage are always reviewed during an FDA GLP inspection. As building space is put on a premium, storage space becomes costly and cumbersome. A humidity- and temperature-controlled space is required for your paper records, or the paper sticks and becomes illegible for inspection. Many GLP firms are scanning historical documents or paying premiums for third-party storage. The return on investment for a 21 CFR Part 11-compliant electronic record system pays for itself and begins to produce profit in the short term.

I would advise off-site, or possibly cloud-based and out-of-state catastrophic-data backup, which is still a fraction of the cost for physical paper storage. Here is the deal: FDA and the US government, in general, are going to require electronic-data submission. Currently, FDA strongly advises electronic application and certification for regulated product submission. I fully appreciate reviewing toxicity and tissue studies for the science aspect however the process of test-article discovery and characterization drives me.

It seems that GLP for FDA is more of a reactionary, domestic self-compliance program area. This means that FDA will get to your firm every few years unless there is a major complaint or significant animal die-off (test subjects). I have observed that a proactive approach is far more productive and necessary, but I am just an ant in the grand scheme of things. I somehow do not grasp the need to flounder and waffle while health-care products may be stopped in their tracks for not proving effectiveness or the toxicity outweighs the benefit. Nonclinical GLP, in my mind, is a key aspect of human clinical trials and should be provided robust and current guidance. I am not only talking about equipment validation or animal maintenance but am also including ICH and global quality processes and standards for GLP. I followed the GLP FDA compliance program for every audit I conducted. I looked at test articles for all the FDA centers represented at the GLP operation and consistently reviewed more than the minimum amount of GLP studies requested. I figured, if the FDA will not be back for two years, I am going to "vertically probe" the entire operation and provide FDA-issued guidance when necessary. The GLP job is too important to let veer off the regulated path. FDA's oversight job is too important to just let it fail.

Most GLP firms service health-product firms in multiple BIMO program areas. Many different chemical entities and biological test articles may be on study at one GLP firm. If there is a quality-process violation, it may affect many products and projects. Most of the GLP firms I inspected contracted toxicity and necropsy tissue studies to third-party operations. I have not seen an FDA inspection assignment for a third-party GLP firm, but I am sure they get inspected. The advanced BIMO GLP class I attended went into great detail and hands-on viewing of wet and dry tissue slides (multiple species). There were no inspections in the Dallas District for this type of GLP review. We could have used two weeks of this type of training, but less is more, right? Wrong, it takes toxicologists a lifetime to learn tissue specification and disease-state recognition. One week is not going to even scratch the surface.

The next area to look at is Bioequivalence. Bioequivalence is one of the most challenging of the BIMO program areas. Many bioequivalence firms get into regulatory oversight issues because it is so difficult to juggle highly sensitive equipment, patient drug samples, protocol adherence, strict timelines, biostatistics, electronic system validation and reproducibility, and regulatory compliance. One missed or erroneous starting calculation for these bioequivalence projects will not be accepted by the center. Incomplete study validation during a bioequivalence projects may produce million dollar mistakes for your stakeholders. I cannot tell you how many times I have issued a 483 observation form knowing the reviewed bioequivalence study would have to be thrown out and redone.

The center (CDER DSI) does not give any wiggle room to bioequivalence firms, nor does it cut any review corners when on site. Many of my international trips were for bioequivalence inspections. I worked with some of the most knowledgeable and professional individuals the FDA has. I often used the opportunities to increase my technical knowledge of LC/MS/MS from the experts. Most of the bioequivalence training field investigators get is on the job.

Many of my big cases involved bioequivalence inspections. The bioequivalence industry appears to try very hard to build compliance into their system. It takes many man-hours and highly technical staff to run a medium- to large-scale bioequivalence operation. The big drug pharma companies see generic and new delivery system. Gel tabs and fast delivery system drugs are flooding the market, and bioequivalence is what it takes to get these reformulated drugs to market. There are abbreviated inspection approaches and abridged report writing submission; however, I did not use these approaches very often. The investigators have report-writing options for no-action-indicated inspections (NAI) for all BIMO program areas (PDUFA for drugs and MDUFA for devices). I felt that a full report with exhibits was the best way for the Review Division to conduct their business. I felt that clinical trials are too important to just say, "All is well, and on to the next inspection." The work FDA does is critical to all of us, and there should be no shortcuts. One bioequivalence firm services multiple BIMO program areas and many different pharmaceutical firms. If there is a quality process violation, it may affect many test articles and projects. If process validation sounds familiar, it's because I'm stressing the need for updated compliance programs, including a section for LC/MS/MS review. Industry will take cues from this guidance.

FDA should put out more industry-specific guidance for the bioequivalence program area. Industry constantly requests more guidance from FDA. FDA consistently releases bioequivalence guidance that begs more questions from industry rather than actually providing useful scientific applications. With regard to my work in the bioequivalence program area, I followed the compliance program and assisted the center expert when possible. I tried to learn from each BIMO inspection and build upon previous experience. I feel confident in my abilities to review bioequivalence from a field investigator standpoint. I do not feel confident from a reviewer's standpoint in the bioequivalence area, but I will continue to work at it. Even within the FDA bioequivalence team, there are always great discussions and scientific debates. Biostatistics calculation models, laboratory equipment technical parameters, and sensitivity are some of the most debated bioequivalence topics.

I observed firms using wide-tolerance specificity ranges of 10 percent or even 15 percent margin of error. These same firms are using the latest LC/MS/MS equipment capable of less than 1 or 2 percent error and sensitivity at the molecular level. You can literally drive a tugboat through 15 percent margin of error. Set your standards near the output range of your equipment if possible and no more than 5 percent error in order to build reproducibility into your validated test methods. I have also observed data manipulation and falsification that put into question every project ever done by the offending firm. FDA has highly skilled professionals working in the field. These FDA DSI pharmacologists and doctors will find your cut corners and validation violations. I have encountered many bioequivalence project violations by simply asking the right questions. Usually, firm employees want to tell you what the bioequivalence study problems are, and you have to listen.

Field investigators are trained to listen when you speak and verify with data validation. FDA expects 21 CFR Part 11-compliant data systems for a reason. Every keystroke and entry is tracked and time/date stamped. My inspection team would routinely request the audit trail of the entire study period for e-records from the firm's IT staff. If we were provided with a CD, we would check much of the data-correction entries and original entry to clinical-site source documentation. I cannot tell you how many times I observed that the corrected value did not match the source data and had to be changed back to the original entry. If a project is data locked, the data-correction process is that much more complicated. The point is, FDA investigators will find your deficiencies and you will then have to deal with damage control. The stressful call to your affected customers will heat up as questions mount. Multiple verification steps for each process, with expert QA review, is a step in the right direction but does not insure that FDA will still find the gap in your armor.

Sponsor monitor inspections were far and few between for me until my last two years in the agency. The FDA decided it was time to actually do routine inspections on sponsor and monitor firms. Before 2008, I had not had a routine sponsor or monitor inspection; they had all been for-cause complaint inspections. In fact, most of the sponsor audits were combination audits. I was there to inspect the Clinical Investigator, who was also the sponsor and manufacturer. There are many personalized-medicine Clinical Investigators in Houston that are all-in-one. I am not sure if FDA chooses firms randomly or by a two-year timetable; however, firms should be inspected based on output. Output is the volume of human clinical trials ongoing and the amount of clinical sites in a clinical trial. A logical biostatistical approach based on science and risk should be used for determining FDA BIMO inspections. I was not able to apply logic as an FDA team member because the grunts do what they're told, not what they think is logical. I am happy to apply logic to my thought process now as an ex-FDA investigator. I am not stating that FDA conducts business wrong, because the direction and final outcome are not wrong.

The US food supply and health-care system were top of the global line in the twentieth century. FDA now needs to move into the twenty-first century. I am trying to interject efficiency and effectiveness into the equation – is that too much to ask from my tax dollars? The FDA is a great organization that is very small with a family feel to it. Just as I cannot tell my parents, "Hey, you did things absolutely wrong raising me." FDA was my life, and now in hindsight, it is very clear, so consider this my addition to the big suggestion box. I have no illusions that my words will affect any change. I am an outsider now, but maybe some of you out there will write to Congress or conduct your clinical trials with a few of my recommendations added to your procedures. Global health is our mission, and it must succeed for our longevity. Sponsors have a great responsibility to build compliance into every test-article project. FDA's responsibility is to ensure that every test article approved for market is effective and safe.

Sponsors have an obligation to train Clinical Investigators and clinical staff human clinical-trial protocol requirements and project expectations. In my humble opinion an open dialogue should be encouraged during investigator meetings and throughout the study period. During BIMO inspection discussions with many Clinical Investigators, they have stated that portions of the protocol were not in line with current medical practice. I have also recommended that protocol worksheets or tools may be used to capture patient evaluations and source data. These work sheets could be shared with the sponsor for implementation approval. Sponsors should be providing all the necessary tools for their expensive trials to succeed and build compliance into the protocol. Very simple clinic staff procedures may be required at every step of the protocol with QA follow-up. The only possible outcomes are patient safety and compliant data when enhanced regulatory procedures are implemented. End point efficacy data points must be captured in clinical trial source documentation to ensure test article biostatistical proofs. Sponsors must also ensure that serious adverse events (SAE) are reported in a timely manner, including IRB SAE submissions. Many data-capturing tools and flowcharts may be utilized to enhance protocol compliance. The seemingly trivial initiatives and detail orientation add to compliance in your global health initiatives.

Take the accountants and business aspect out of this equation. Sponsors have individuals' lives in their hands. Make sure your sponsors are putting the patients or test subject before your bottom line. A full book should be written for each program area and import. If your project is effective and safe, it may go global and your return on investment will be compensated. Your regulatory diligence will produce a quality product. Let's talk global shop now!

CHAPTER 5

International BIMO Inspections

FDA'S INSPECTION PROGRAM provides for inspection of international clinical sites, manufacturers, and other regulated entities. International inspections will always be necessary to protect and serve the US public health. Imports and imported products are a fact of life and global progress. FDA will always have to send investigators out for international inspections. The United States consumes and uses more imported products with growth in every program area annually. I would recommend FDA international travel to any willing to get on the plane. FDA needs more able and willing field investigators ready to cross the big ponds. I was willing to conduct many more FDA international inspections, but never will. FDA must enhance security before requesting more foreign trips from the field staff.

For several weeks at a time, an experienced FDA investigator, or team of investigators are sent on a globetrotting series of inspections at usually great cost. These international inspections appear to require more communication/ cohesion between the centers and trip planners. In my humble opinion the BIMO international trips are not cost-effective and lack logistics. I am positive that if an FDA investigator travels to Italy for a clinical-investigator BIMO inspection for CBER, then possibly, CDER has an inspection for a different test article or bioequivalence in the same country. Right now, field investigators may start a BIMO in Canada then fly to Italy over the weekend and end up in Argentina the last week of travel. You tell me how this makes any logistical sense and I will follow your leadership.

If at any point the investigator gets stuck in transit, injured, sick, or volcanoes go off, and you cannot fly out, then what? The rest of your great FDA itinerary sent from the center is disrupted. I have made a few of these multi-country trips and hit snags in my travel. It gets irritating quickly, and happy thoughts of getting paid extra for the travel ground you. With fuel costs and disruption in flight-service scenarios, logic should dictate that FDA send the field investigator to one country for two or three weeks to do cross-center inspections. I have suggested this to the highest FDA authority with mediocre response at best. I was told very early in my FDA tenure that I had to throw logic out the door and "think government." I struggled to the last day with trying to "think government" with the burden of waste and loss of vital resources. Going green should not be a catch phrase but a way of life, period (recycle, reuse, and reduce waste)!

Why pay a travel-service provider to track and charge you when not so long ago, the FDA had a travel provider that tracked and helped us for free on our travel. Simple, cost-effective measures can save millions, but you have to stop "thinking government." I am very capable of making my flight arrangements and hotel reservations, thanks; you already gave me the government credit card. You tracked my financial statements and validated my public trust. GovTrip is a poorly designed, tedious, time-gauging computer-based travel software. GovTrip and the other tracking systems cost millions, and the voucher fees are depleting valuable limited resources.

I would like to know who designed the GovTrip software; it is simply wasteful. Why can't the government have a cost-free travel system? Because "Think Government" waste is pervasive at every level of the organization. I own a travel portal, and I make money on any travel I take for personal and business travel. If a simple mind like mine can profit from travel, then surely the FDA can also profit from any travel it mandates. The current system has FDA paying twenty or thirty dollars per travel voucher. If the traveler has a problem or has to call the travel provider (happens all the time), a service fee is added to the travel voucher. The FDA is being charged triple for errors caused by the travel system. It makes no sense. I would like to sell FDA my three hundred-dollar travel service provided by Rovia so the organization could make millions in travel usage. If many globally recognized organizations and franchises are signed up, I am sure they can handle another four thousand or so FDA staff to the Rovia rolls. Maybe the FDA can model the Rovia system to make its own system.

Why do contractors with hackable systems facilitate sensitive-government travel arrangements? If hackers can infiltrate US government top-secret contractors with robust cyber secure systems, a contractor travel system is vulnerable. FDA travelers go into hostile international territories, and travel itineraries should be secure with the most-advanced cybersecurity. I do not know if the current FDA travel contractors utilize the best for FDA field staff when on travel, because I have been in the field under fire and I was not secure.

I started traveling in May of 2003 and traveled at least twice a year until December 2009, conducting approximately twenty international inspections during those seven years. FDA sent me to Canada, Europe, Mexico, and South America during my international travel duty. FDA provides investigators with international travel training, which is more like an etiquette refresher on how not to act when representing the FDA. The class is not program specific, and you do not learn until too late that you now have double-work and half the normal time to complete it. You are told that interpreters slow the process down with misinterpretations and lost-in-translation moments. You are not told just how much of your time you will be training your interpreter. It helps to already know a few languages and have experience traveling within the countries you are sent to. Trying not to act like the rude, obnoxious American on tour is very important for succeeding on your international trips for business or pleasure. I have made many friends and respected colleagues from my many trips, including trips that resulted in a 483 observation issuance. FDA investigators are basically invited guests in a foreign country with little regulatory authority. You must be an ambassador of good will and an ultimate champion for patient safety. These individuals may never see another FDA investigator or worse when they do have another inspection have to explain how terrible the last visit went.

FDA has no authority to issue a 482, Notice of Inspection, in a foreign country, so that is the first big difference in the inspection mind-set. The firms know that you are out of your element until the records and the request for comments on protocol deviations come out; then their tone changes quickly. I enjoyed surprising international firms with my language skills and adaptability to any situation. The level of background-investigation technique required to conduct a foreign inspection is no less than six or seven years of experience. FDA should not be so quick to send out very green investigators who cannot adapt to any situation. The foreign-industry perception will be that FDA is a pushover. FDA should not rush investigators to the Foreign Service call because the results may be disastrous. I have heard many new investigators come back from a "volunteer" foreign trip and saying they will never take another trip, not understanding it is mandatory.

I cannot stress the need for foreign inspections with an increase in BIMO audits. FDA needs to train this new crew more if they want to speed this process up. I felt shortchanged on FDA training but flew by the seat of my pants and came back home every time with more world knowledge. Management makes foreign travel unpleasant by mandates and lack of security involved with international travel. The grueling multicounty inspections have to be rethought and evaluated by upper management. Volunteers are needed for international trips, and there are far too many third and fourth requests from the center. District management must mandate and pick a traveler if no one volunteers. Some international trips have requests from the host-country health department for participation in the FDA inspection. FDA, in some cases, also requests informal meetings with host-country health agencies.

I have been asked to wear many hats on an international trip. I recall presenting in Buenos Aires, Argentina, to the director generals and doctors of the Administración Nacional de Medicamentos, Alimentos y Tecnología Médica (ANMAT) (*http://www.anmat.gov.ar/principal.asp*) and feeling like the small fry. They listened to my Spanish translation of FDA guidance and field-investigator responsibilities. I probably left them with more questions than answers. I was glad to try and give them a simplified perspective of BIMO work and test-article preapproval. They had all read the FDA CPGMs and 21 CFR regulations written in English. I attempted to translate some of the technical BIMO regulatory concepts and answer as many questions as I possibly could. Reflecting back on my presentation for ANMAT, I would have stated a few BIMO concepts more effectively. Patient safety, protocol adherence, and test article accountability are the triangle base to build from. The guidance, CPGM, and regulations are now available in Spanish. In Argentina, all the field investigators are medically trained or doctors. They are not a very big organization, but ANMAT does a great service for Argentina's public health. The ANMAT directors had many bioequivalence questions that were very difficult to answer because of the technical Spanish translation. I did my best to provide Tex-Mex Spanish responses for some of the questions discussed. I later privately apologized to my departed grandparents. I silently vowed to learn technical Spanish in order to explain bioequivalence. I have already mentioned that when FDA investigators conduct bioequivalence inspections, the center Review Division is part of the on-site inspection team and does most of the technical-record review (Pharm D, PhD, and MD).

I have gone to Canada many times for bioequivalence work and sample collections. The Canadian health investigators have shadowed one of my inspections; however, I did not meet with them very much in my many trips to Canada.

The Brazilian National Health Surveillance Agency (Anvisa, established in January 1999) worked with me on one of my two trips to Brazil. Many current national health organizations are less than ten years old and use FDA's template to build on their country's regulatory oversight. More BIMO guidance for industry will also provide useful information for other national health organizations. FDA is intent on reorganizing and restructuring with little time left for leading the global health mission. During this restructuring period, the FDA is leaning toward established European Medicines Agency (EMA) standards and ICH guides. FDA will take a passenger seat to this global mission if they lean too far over to the Atlantic side. My point here is that FDA's global health partners need enhanced guidance from FDA outside the normal channels of public forum. The compliance strategy is a good resource for other national health organizations to follow.

The FDA transparency initiative will help global health organizations by providing a 483 citation database by year. This will help track and trend the FDA focus areas that will translate to ongoing human clinical research globally. Health organizations want proof that FDA model is working with numbers to match effectiveness. FDA-study audit inspections' ratio to the entire amount of ongoing clinical trials is very low at 1 percent or less. It is very difficult to establish effectiveness with such low numbers to evaluate. Today it can be said that you have to add up five years' worth of BIMO inspections to get a significant sampling of 483 trends in clinical research. The problem with this method is, it is a day late and a dollar short of effecting national self-compliance. I have heard many managers state that with the high demand for foreign travel, the FDA will have to rely on domestic self-compliance as a working model. I am shocked to hear such talk because as a field investigator, I find many "hot" domestic cases. In my mind, settling for less than 1 percent domestic inspections is not acceptable, considering the amount of issues still observed. I feel that FDA should review 20 or 30 percent study review. FDA should review at minimum 15 percent study review because FDA expects IRBs to review this amount. Lead by example and get compliance or settle for less-than-adequate compliance. Most of the BIMO center managers understand the ration of international BIMO inspections is much greater than FDAs domestic inventory. Like many other industries lost to out-sourcing, clinical trials are conduced exponentially more out of this country as compared to within the continental US. The FDA in this light will have to increase the amount of international BIMO inspections. How will the FDA pay for this necessity? The US Congress holds the purse strings and international BIMO regulatory concerns should not dwindle. If FDA replicated its force (force multiply) by training other countries' health organizations to conduct FDA business with memorandums of understanding (MOU), less money could be used to travel with more inspections completed. The EMA should have an MOU if their model is similar to FDA's. The advent of all-electronic review should alleviate the need for more international review. I may be oversimplifying the issues with training monies and bringing foreign inspectors to US training facilities. Host nations can send their inspectors for knowledge sharing and training with justifiable benefits to the host nations' public health. FDA can also video link for training, as I suggested earlier in the training section. Innovative options are scarce, and the old way of doing business is ingrained into the government model. For the short term, FDA will try to increase international inspections in all program areas.

Food inspections will be the emphasis program with monies earmarked for food inspections only. FDA has historically conducted more BIMO, drug, device, and biologic international inspections. This model is changing fast with international food inspection projected to be over five hundred. FDA cannot do virtual food inspections, so this is a positive step in the right direction. FDA is consistently adding to the imports staff for more import coverage. This is also a much-needed direction because imports can catch so much more noncompliant/unsafe food products from entering the market. FDA tries to lead cases that clearly should be handed over to US Customs for immediate detention and destruction. There is no room for competition between agencies.

A seamless overlap is needed for cost-effective regulatory compliance. International inspections and import surveillance are very important parts of the market safety net. FDA has been stationing managers and support staff in many host-nation capitals. I am not sure if field investigators will ever be requested to join the established offices with the budget constraints. The field investigators are the last to be told anything, so I am not sure what the plans are. I do know that many of us have had rough travel experiences with very little feedback from other investigators. There should be a forum for all international travelers to review previous international travel incidents in order to make informed decisions on safe travel destinations. Some FDA investigators have been stuck in the Iceland volcano eruption that stopped travel across the Atlantic. I want to know that I am not the only magnet for disaster and laugh with my fellow travelers at the world we live in while back in the office safe and sound.

FDA keeps a database of international-travel incidents. I hope one day the managers feel the transparency bug and provide this information to the field travelers. My last official international travel for FDA was in Mexico. Let me say I am Mexican American, and I used to love going to Mexico. Cabrito in Monterrey, Mexico, with their local Indio beer, is the best. It may be years before I go back to Mexico. On December 17, 2009, in Cuernavaca, Mexico, I was blocks away from where the biggest drug lord (at the time) in the world was taken down and in harm's way. Grenades were going off and automatic-weapons' fire could be heard very clearly. The armored personnel tanks were rolling in while sponsor representatives and I tried to get a taxi back to the hotel, which was five miles away. A Mexican soldier pointed his M-16 machine gun at us because we went down the "wrong road," so we turned around. It took us hours to get back to the hotel that was on lockdown. I did not feel safe, and my life was in danger. I asked to be recalled for my personal safety, but my request was denied. I was on the bottom of the FDA food chain but never had I felt so expendable. I will always remember my experience and the loss of state department lives one month after I returned home. The ultimate sacrifice was made by those brave civil servants, who would not change their lives for the sake of a drug war being waged at and within our borders. I hope for a more secure and safe future for all of us. You cannot run a business in the midst of a dangerous war because of the randomness of war.

I should have known back in October of 2002 when I took my orientation to international inspection class that security was not the main concern during your trip planning. I state this because the 1999 *Guide to International Inspections and Travel* dedicates five pages out of one hundred and seventeen to security. Safety for the field investigator is more of an afterthought for FDA in my experience. I have spoken with many fellow FDA international travelers with similar stories of great escapes and near-death scenarios. I was not the first or the last to escape by the skin of my shorts out of harm's way. The day I left, there were police stationed at every street and the whole city was on lockdown. The Mexican authorities kept finding bodies of the people who took the protection money for this drug lord. I kissed the Texas ground when I finally made it back home. I told myself never again would I put my life in danger for anyone who did not value my life.

Life is too short and precious to die just when your young family has been started. I cannot help my family or play with my two beautiful babies if I am six feet under. The worst part for me about this whole experience is that my district management all the way up the chain did not acknowledge the seriousness of my situation, with no e-mails or calls of concern until years later. I understand everyone is busy, but when the life of one of the team's members is in danger, the whole mission is in danger. Without the worker ants, the nest dies or has nothing more to do. Senior management better get their act together because the most-qualified FDA civil servants are jumping ship because of management issues. I will say this many times. I did not leave the FDA; I left the FDA management. I was not willing to go to the union or fight my way through to end up bitter and be crushed. *I will continue the BIMO mission and make a difference in my field of choice.* I will not be distracted by sidebar issues and personal-glory projects by managers who are not qualified to lead. I have looked up the backgrounds of many upper managers, and they do not have consistent warning letters or actionable cases in the full FDA spectrum. If I have more regulatory actions than you do and you try to lead me with your bold, new directives, I will laugh. You can change the name for an agenda or busy work, but it will still be pointless and time-consuming. If you managers would just let the field staff do their job, maybe some proposed goals would get accomplished. The old ways of giving assignments worked for the worker bee investigators and for the rest, mandate what they do until they prove trust worthy to complete the mission.

Congress continues to tighten the budget due to our borrowing money to run the expanded government. Congress also continues to mandate more international travel from FDA. It would seem more logical to enhance import surveillance with advanced detection for cost-effectiveness. Travel to foreign destinations always has inherent risk factors and unanticipated events. The benefit from knowledge sharing and regulatory guidance explanation is a priceless return on the international travel investment. I am not stating FDA has to stop international travel, because that is unwise. FDA must evolve and become proactive out in the field. The import division will now have to mandate that field investigators add international travel to the position description. The import division makes up almost half of FDA staff with inspectors and investigators. The import investigators will have to add international travel to the list of things to do. For now, domestic field staff bear the brunt of international travel. The new hires will, hopefully, be ready to fly out in a few more years. Sending out individuals that are not ready for the compressed timetable and language issues is counterproductive. The international firms will know on the way that the investigator is inexperienced. Investigators with years of field experience in the program area considered for travel and a firm grasp of regulatory compliance concepts should be selected to travel. The FDA will, in some cases, have to send investigators with limited field experience out for the crash course.

I became a more efficient investigator after a few years of international travel; you are forced to elevate your skills. I suggest traveling and would recommend international travel for those that are ready. I will never forget the culture and food on my many travels. I will, most of all, not forget the professional regulators and clinic study staff I worked with over the years. I still get e-mails and contact calls from many former customers. I hope to continue my international travels on the contract side. Multisite and multinational human clinical trials are the future of global health care. It is better to have a broad-spectrum population sample included in human clinical trials for complete biostatistical sampling. The cultural exchange is knowledge you cannot get from a book. It takes thinking outside the box every day you are on an international trip. Three weeks of travel used to fly by in an instant. Now that I have a family, three weeks is an eternity. I do not mind two-week travel or even weekly travel. I have noticed more two-week FDA international trips in 2010-2011. I knew I would not take another trip for FDA after the Mexico event. I forgive, but I will never forget the danger my family was in. When I am in harm's way, so is my family.

FDA management understands and struggles with completing the public health mission but must mandate trip selections. Many of the twenty- and thirty-year veterans are not so eager to volunteer for three-week trips for various reasons. FDA has had to take away many incentives provided to international travelers. Business class flight time has been increased out of many countries' availability. Security is an afterthought more than a process. Shrinking per diem and hotel allowance will keep volunteers at bay. The biggest roadblock hindering many three-week trips is the travel within travel every weekend. I explained to my managers that international travel is already a mad dash to get there; throw in travel on every weekend and the equation turns into a nightmare.

I did not volunteer for trips that had extra-continental travel, but I did have to take a few of these trips. I do not mind a little travel within a country or surrounding two-hundred-mile radius. You ask too much of a traveler to be packing and unpacking every five days for three weeks. You can never really get your stuff back into your luggage the same as when you first packed the bags. I can also tell you that having to pay out of pocket for your clothes to be washed in a foreign country is ridiculous and stinky. I have paid hundreds of dollars in having my clothes washed at local establishments other than the eye-gouging hotels. I would have spent thousands of dollars using every hotel's laundry service. There are so many reasons not to travel that finding a good reason to volunteer for these trips becomes a federal project. I will tell you that because the FDA does not give out real bonuses and pay raises that many field investigators volunteer for the extra money associated with saving money on an international trip. I tried to get much of my international travel in early thinking I would be at the bottom of the list for mandate travel. Wrong answer, I became a workhorse go-to guy for more travel expectations. My plan backfired, and I put the brakes on real quick after eight long years. Did management ever thank us for making the district/region and the agency look like they were performing? They received their bonus and expected more with less for another big payout. Thanks for no thanks; you woke me up after standing on my back. Did I mention the five-year pay freeze?

I have recently observed international firms receiving warning letters and multiple-item 483 forms. If this current warning-letter trend continues, the blame may fall on lack of regulatory guidance. The core mission of FDA is to protect the US public from harmful health products. Sending FDA field investigators to where the products are manufactured and undergo human clinical trials is one of the only ways to accomplish the core mission. Ensuring that field investigators are proficient for the task and seasoned investigators stay engaged will be the challenge. I did my best to impart knowledge and mentor the new hires and state inspectors. I know it will not be long before the new hires I took out on inspections will be shuffled off into the international cadre. I let each of them know how intense and detail oriented international inspection can be. I tried to explain my thought and stepwise CPGM approach for each type of inspection we conducted. You cannot take a new hire out on a foreign inspection because only GS-12 journeyman-grade investigators are allowed out of the country. Some of the Dallas District investigators are not receiving their step increases, which will delay the amount of investigators available for the international team. For the two- and three-year new hires, it will take them at least three years on the domestic side. The basic concepts of FDA must be ingrained into the new hires so they will be ready for the grueling task of three-week foreign travel. If the new hires conduct mainly food-program work internationally, they will do well. Congressional mandates increased the amount of international food program work exponentially, and the import division has enhanced operations.

FDA will have to think outside the box if congressional mandates for international travel are to be met. Congress must also understand that it is not only the amount of funds that ensure successful international travel but it is also about proficient field investigators. I have faith that FDA field staff will answer the challenge; they always do. Upper management tries to keep the bar set at levels that can be met. I would estimate that FDA conducts two hundred BIMO program inspections internationally.

How many ongoing clinical trials worldwide are for test articles trying to enter the US market? You cannot really understand the numbers because even if I stated that there are one hundred thousand trials ongoing for entry into the US market, it would be an understatement. FDA is going to have to increase domestic inspections while mandating many more trips to India and China. I have not traveled to the Far East in my personal or professional excursions. I know it is only a matter of time before I make the twenty-plus-hour flight to our global market partners. Many of the current BIMO trips are for China and India due to high volume of ongoing current human clinical trials. Informed consent and human-subject rights would be my main review aspects during a regulatory compliance audit in any foreign country. I did not change my focus areas or distinguish between domestic and international FDA inspections. The same 21 CFR rules applied to every international site, and all the clinicians should understand this concept. Sponsors and monitors need to educate the clinic staff and Principal Investigators, including FDA expectations minus the fear mongering. FDA is not going abroad to beat up firms. FDA goes abroad to ensure regulatory compliance minus the politics and personal feelings about individual cultures. FDA trains international investigators to interact with foreign governments and firm employees. Strong-arm tactics are not part of the training, and on the contrary, FDA international cadre trainers request that investigators explain each and every 483 observation.

Field investigators are requested to discuss any findings early in the inspection for comments and clarification before the closeout. I would always follow this policy so that clinic staff had plenty of time to respond or propose corrective actions. The goal should always be compliance, not "Let's make an example of this international company." My international inspection closeout discussions with a 483 issuance were always half-a-day sessions. I wanted to make sure none of the items were lost in translation or unclear. I tried to give every firm the opportunity to propose corrective action and regulatory compliance guidance. I did not issue very many international BIMO 483 observation forms during my time at FDA, but I gave many verbal-discussion items and used my regulatory discretion. Patient safety was not compromised, and for the most part, administrative issues can be amended. I did not consider myself to be a pushover or easy. I tried to be fair and encouraged regulatory compliance.

In my experience, foreign firms expected professionalism and feedback in the form of guidance. It always seemed there was a daily closeout meeting with the Principal Investigators and staff. Domestically I did not meet with the Principal Investigators every day during an inspection unless requested. If I had observations to discuss or serious problems were encountered, then the face time would increase drastically. During my international travels, I encountered very knowledgeable and capable staff conducting clinical trials or bioequivalence laboratory work. The problems usually didn't occur when sponsors trained and provided clinical sites with all the tools necessary to successfully complete a clinical trial in regulatory compliance. Monitoring is a vital process to ensure regulatory QA and protocol compliance for every project. I will repeat this thought process to every sponsor and CRO. Monitoring clinical trials ensures regulatory compliance when the auditors go in for site initiation training and continue to make regular QA visits. Many sponsors and monitors get caught up on what a regular visit is. There is a statistical method for conducting clinical trials, and so you may use a statistical method to figure out what is normal. It does not matter what phase your project is in; the model will not change because special consideration and patient safety are critical in every phase of the project. My team can help develop the amount of monitoring required to achieve success in every project your company works on.

I will continue to collaborate with global health project sponsors on-site or via remote access. I do not wish to keep my service domestic because the United States is not an isolated, self-sustaining island. The United States is a melting-pot market with individuals and goods from every corner of the earth. I will continue to partner with emerging markets in South America, Europe, China, and India. I hope my words here will give insight into the FDA thought process and guide your effective health-care projects to a successful market share. The regulations have been established to ensure safe and effective products are introduced into the global market. The globalization of the regulations with EMA and other regulatory bodies will ensure that compliance in one country ensures compliance in the collective body. We should work smarter, not necessarily harder. I believe in good work ethics, and the BIMO program area is for hard, detail-oriented workers with a passion to provide health care. You have to love this work because compassionate health care can be a demanding endeavor.

Making a difference in global health and making money are a few of the motivators for this business. I hope that making a difference for global health is your main motivation with asset compensation as a result. I will continue to make global health my primary mission and passion. FDA field investigators that go on foreign inspections become a one-person army with multiple tasks to complete simultaneously.

Depending on the amount of study subjects, primary end points, length of trial, and complexity of test article, five days can be an eternity or lifetime. I cannot tell you how many times the site has stated to me that one week is not enough time for the amount of study subjects to review. I routinely reviewed all the study subjects in each foreign trial because that was the goal I set for every international BIMO review. I explained to each site Clinical Investigator; they might not see FDA for a long time. The bioequivalence firms knew that the amount of work they put out directly related to the amount of times they would be audited by FDA. All the bioequivalence firms I inspected had been through many FDA inspection teams. The bioequivalence inspection teams consist of the field investigator and Division of Scientific Investigations (DSI) CDER field staff.

The international bioequivalence inspections are conducted just like the domestic inspections. International bioequivalence firms go through vendor audits, qualifications, EMA review, FDA audits, and their own federal mandate inspections. FDA should provide bioequivalence guidance for domestic and international firms to expand on enhanced scientific methods. I have observed too many foreign firms react surprised and confused when we read the 483 observations. This could have language-translation factors, or current guidance leaves too much to the imagination. If FDA decided to open a comment forum to the bioequivalence field worldwide, the center would need to dedicate extra staff for going through legitimate regulatory concerns. Most international bioequivalence firms want to take you out for dinner so they can continue discussions on FDA regulatory strategy and worst-case-scenario stories. We were instructed not to be rude or turn down hospitality, but I always offered to pay my own tab. The cultural exchange around the dinner table builds bridges and solidifies trust between global health partners. I have so many cherished pictures, maps, postcards, clothing items, and collectibles from around the globe (all items I purchased with personal funds). Every country has unique solutions to global health problems that can be implemented and built on. The FDA has laid out the road map to success; staying on regulatory course from cradle to grave for your test article is the desired outcome, and QA is the solution.

If you contract my QA team for your projects, we will review 100 percent of the study subjects to ensure patient safety and regulatory compliance with the US market. TradeStone QA will use the methodologies listed in this book, which are only scratching the regulatory surface of our combined fifty-plus years' field, center, and supervisory FDA experience. I would not venture too far into any project without a core team of well-connected individuals who are able to speak and interpret FDA language. The FDA language is complex in the simple and general statements the centers provide, which are open to interpretation with great expectations. I want to help your projects stay no action indicated (NAI) or, worst case, voluntary action indicated (VAI). I will not allow my contracted firms to conduct official-action-indicated (OAI) work because failure is not an option in my program. We are all human and make mistakes, in order to learn from them.

OAI work means that you deliberately put subjects' lives in jeopardy and a multimillion-dollar health project may be put on hold. On that note, let's take a walk down the OAI aisle and review a few of the major cases I worked, without the names, of course, to protect the regulatory challenged firms out there. I do not take pride in issuing 483 observation forms; however, I am proud of any lives I may have saved by preventing harmful products entering the US/global market.

CHAPTER 6

Official-Action-Indicated (OAI) Work

O FFICIALLY, EACH FDA inspection conducted receives one of three outcome classifications. These are commonly known as NAI (No Action Indicated,) VAI (Voluntary Action Indicated,) and OAI (Official Action Indicated.) NAI and VAI classifications usually do not result in FDA correspondence or actions, while OAI typically means at least a Warning Letter will result. Most of the OAI work I have presented to FDA compliance has been for Clinical Investigators, bioequivalence laboratories, and IRBs. For the Clinical Investigator (CI)/Principal Investigator (PI) inspections, the deficiency trend continues to be with following the protocol and serious-adverse-event reporting.

The key points here are hiring knowledgeable, clinically trained, and credentialed staff. Principal Investigators should also go over the source documentation real time or at least weekly. I have seen good clinical sites go the wrong direction due to employee overturn or other retention issues. It is very difficult to train staff midway through a clinical protocol, especially if that staff is already working on three different projects. Just think about that: managing CRO supervisors and directors when you do not meet sponsor expectations look to increase the staff you have or continue to fail. Principal Investigators make sure your study staff is qualified to conduct clinical trials. Principal Investigators just because you are invincible and can multi-task that does not mean your staff have the same constitution.

If the study patients are treated by non-study-trained staff, make sure all staff know how to document treatment visits and data-capture procedures. Using a study flowchart and data-capture tools are necessary to ensure protocol compliance. Building quality into your system and working to retain your staff are part of your job. If the data-capture system for source documents is electronic, you can easily mandate study entry-data points for non-study patient-care providers. I can help you with retaining your staff and your clinical trials, if you let me. We humans work most efficient when happy and healthy. If you want biobots, you better get in line; they cost a million dollars each and cannot think outside the box, so you still may have to do some of the work.

I am not going to give away the farm here; so you will have to contact our team for the technical issues concerning the FDA, 21 CFR, and guidance. I am not even scratching the surface of my twelve-year service and combined fifty-plus years with the team. An all-inclusive FDA book series could fill up volumes like a hundred-book encyclopedia (try our Library of Congress). We have much to discuss with the global health community and US public. I am not trying to make you like FDA investigators or become one. I am trying to state the need for public awareness and protection. Nanny state regulations are very cost-prohibitive and wasteful. FDA needs to regulate internal agency waste and external import fraud as focus points. We can do more with less if wasteful practice is taken out of the equation.

The current FDA electronic-data systems can track, trend, and report what each investigator is working on or has completed. Management insists that field investigators make a monthly agenda. This is a worthless exercise because every day brings changes and adjustments. Managers, pick up your fingers and pull the data out. If the director of investigator branch wants a report on your team's activity, have the system generate a report in seconds and e-mail away. Or better yet, hey, DIB, pull up whatever your heart desires on the data stream and do your job for the field staff. There is too much busy work for the sake of looking busy. The US consumers deserve the best utilization of the tax burden they put in. I am trying to help you get a glimpse of the world FDA regulates and some of the language used to regulate your world. We would like you to get the TradeStone QA team involved with your global health projects as soon as possible because there is much to be done.

Many times Clinical Investigators take on too many projects at one time. It is very difficult to manage faculty positions, regular practice, resident training, and run three or more human clinical trials. I will say this again: you are not superhuman. You have been given a gift to use for healing, not a godlike power. You must rest, be with family, and work hard, of course.

I have given many long 483 observation forms to Clinical Investigators that were over their heads or delegated study control to the wrong CRO. Principal Investigators must review all study entries, adverse events, and test-article accountability real time. You cannot wait a week or two and get to it when time permits. If you do not stay on top of your projects, they will run away from you and come back later to haunt you. So many problems can be fixed early on, but waiting for monitors to discover problems a month later will not provide great results. Clinical Investigators, you have to tend to the farm every day. It is your name on the contracts, and you are ultimately responsible for any violations. It is very easy to delegate responsibilities to another and very difficult to hoe the row in front of you. When you make a contract and an oath to uphold patient safety, FDA expects to verify it. You cannot run a clinical-study site like a standard-care clinic. If a Principal Investigator must delegate patient care responsibility, make sure it is to a well-qualified medical professional. Most of the clinical-investigator warning letters I have on file are for patient-safety violations, informed-consent violations, and data-integrity violations.

Clinical Investigators should partner up with the IRBs and sponsors to ensure compliance is built into the entire clinical-trial system. Sponsors and IRBs can be notified of serious adverse events simultaneously with updates for follow-up resolution. Clinical Investigators have smart phone access or web-link access to patient-care records. With the advent of comprehensive data access there are now very few reasons to fail in your global health projects.

Most of the major cases for Clinical Investigators were in the device BIMO program area. As I mentioned before, device BIMOs generally have less monitoring from CROs, and devices in general have a great deal of regulations to keep track of. Many sponsors for high-risk implantable devices are sending consultants and engineers for each device implantation. This is the best way to ensure and document compliance with protocols and projects. The hands-on, proactive approach will pay off in the end when compliance is the result. Micromanaging a trial and slowing down progress can be a concern, so a delicate monitoring balance must be maintained. I have seen so many ways to build a better mousetrap, so it is now time to help innovate and recommend strategies to get your projects completed. Clinical Investigators and sponsors, I hope you see the value in contracting or conducting QA on all your human clinical-trials projects. I would also recommend qualifying any individuals you consult with to make sure you get your investments worth.

Protocol violations such as inclusion and exclusion violations are viewed as patient-safety problems. Patient-safety issues are taken very seriously by the FDA centers. Patients that do not meet the indication for the test article could be at risk for a serious adverse event. Assuring your study subjects meet inclusion and do not meet exclusion is the most basic aspect of your clinical trial; get it right the first time and every time. Procuring a subject's clinical history and indicating diagnosis are very simple ways to ensure selection compliance. It can be a pain to procure patient records until you include the patient in the equation. Many times, subjects have their records or just need your help to ask for them. Principal Investigators, if the sponsor did not provide all the tools necessary for data capture, make one up and submit it for approval. Many warning letters go out for lack of following the protocol. Ensure your site has every tool necessary for compliant project completion.

Mismanaging the test article and providing the correct dose are also critical issues that can escalate into a regulatory problem. Training clinic staff to be proactive, regulation-aware, and detail-oriented workers is sometimes cost prohibitive or hard to sell. Clinical Investigators, make sure your staff is willing and able to take on your bright ideas and aspirations. I have seen many clinic sites crumble to pieces under the weight of too many projects and not enough qualified staff. I cannot tell you how many research employees have stated to me during an FDA inspection that the Principal Investigator delegated medical work to them or put too many projects on them. Sponsors must also qualify principal Investigators to ensure project completion. Study-staff turnover can be the worst-case scenario for any human clinical trial. The FDA transparency initiative will now give access to all the recent 483 observations listed by year.

Clinical Investigators should take a proactive approach during investigator meetings, to ensure the tools and training necessary are provided to the study site. Clinical Investigators are contracted by the 1572 Statement of Investigator to complete every health-care project with regulatory compliance. I have had principal Investigators explain there were outdated medical practice procedures in the protocol. The sponsor and IRB closeout of your clinical trial is not the times to bring up glaring protocol errors. I have asked many physicians if they brought their concerns to the sponsor. Most stated they did not bring up the observation during the clinical trial period. I have recommended to many Clinical Investigators that they should to be more proactive on upcoming clinical trials. I always recommend taking an active role in streamlining or at least advise on best medical practice available early in the project. Clinical Investigators should take an active role in the protocol development process before the clinical trial starts.

You must tend to the farm every day, or risk losing it. The switch between standard care and human clinical research is like night and day. Clinical Investigators must distinguish between the two, or risk having regulatory issues. Sponsors and monitors share the burden of training every site and preparing for the start-up of the protocol. FDA investigators are required to establish if sponsors provided adequate protocol and regulatory compliance training to clinical investigator sites. If the clinic sites are not adequately trained and provided with every tool necessary for protocol compliance sponsors will share regulatory responsibility. FDA is going to inspect the clinic site and the sponsor for a complete cycle of compliance review. Clinical Investigators must realize that form 1572, Statement of Investigator, they signed in order to conduct human clinical research is binding and includes four parties (PI/MD, sponsor, subject, and FDA). I will state that a well-thought-out 483-response letter can be the difference between a warning letter and VAI. The FDA wants a fifteen-day response time frame in order to consider your response in the final inspection classification. I cannot stress the need to qualify your site and medically trained staff before taking on each project.

Some of my bioequivalence investigations ended with firms closing down and others received warning letters. I have also observed a fair share of notices sent to firms rejecting multiple non-compliant projects. The center decides the final outcomes for these types of actions. When public harm was a possible result in the bioequivalence firm's failure, the FDA review division would get serious. I was chosen to conduct many bioequivalence inspections because of my willingness to lead a team and learn from the senior center members. I may have been the team leader, but the center investigators did the lion's share of the difficult and technical work. I was also able to work with anyone because some of the center teammates were "rigid meanies." I never met a rigid meanie from the center, and I worked with most of the professionals from DSI. I can understand the center's frustration when the district supervisor assigns field investigators not willing or able to lead an advanced team to the bioequivalence inspections. I started conducting bioequivalence inspection as a team member in 2001, and by 2003, I was a team leader. I have led teams that have been responsible for uncovering record/data fraud, technical-equipment violations, employee-training failures, and projects starting off with an erroneous formula. My FDA teams have been responsible for multiple product recalls and market withdrawals and, unfortunately, shutdowns.

I took no pleasure in directly shutting down a business or having people lose their jobs. The United States/world needs more jobs and qualified individuals working at those jobs. It would take years and many different FDA team inspections to finally get to the point of a business closure. FDA does give many chances to industry. First, the firm receives a warning letter and then the firm has to notify all their customers/sponsors whose studies were affected about the warning letter. The FDA centers will not approve studies based on substandard data or firms that are noncompliant with all applicable regulations. I will say that I have sat on the regulatory side of the table, knowing that the firm's project was not going to be approved, and simply stated my 483 list of observations. It is very difficult to redo parts of a protocol or retroactively validate portions of your protocol. "Retroactive" is not a word you want to use as a 483 response to the district. I would put this on every page of this book if I could make sure you respond to every 483 item within the fifteen-day period. Self-compliance is much better than regulatory-mandated compliance. FDA investigators sometimes make mistakes or disregard waivers. FDA investigators have been known to miscalculate and then have to go through the 483 form amendment process or rescind the whole 483 form. I have also helped many Clinical Investigators get erroneous 483 forms amended years after issuance. I am on the side of scientifically based facts, not political will or fiction-derived contrivance. If the FDA is on the wrong side of public health, I will call it out. If I make a mistake, I call it out and say, "I will learn from this and work harder." FDA is not above reproach and, as an organization funded by politics, is fallible. When decisions are based on significant statistically based science, good results happen. When politics and lobby moneybags get involved, you might as well throw science out the window.

Bioequivalence inspections, as I stated before, are the most intense of all the BIMO program inspections. First, you work with a team, and the team members know more about the work than you do. Mass spectrometer LC/MS/MS systems are high-performance quantitation devices used in every phase of the pharmaceutical development process, from discovery to bioequivalence. These systems are used for quantitation and identification applications in protein and peptide analysis, small-molecule analysis in drug metabolism, and pharmacokinetic studies. The Bioequivalence industry must keep their range of acceptance/failure tolerances tight and build in time for project delays. Rushing through project validation with high tolerance ranges, well above equipment detectability range is high school chemistry 101. FDA center experts can see through most of the background noise to find your root cause and project violations. The point here is that it is much easier to spot someone else's failures, especially when that's what you're looking for.

Bioequivalence firms expect validation runs to fail because that is how you learn to correct the process for success. Triple-check with outside eyes, if possible, before you approve your projects. I have witnessed heartache and the wind leave the collective room when the long list of 483 items has been read aloud. I do not want to be the manager to call affected sponsors to advise them of a project hold or reworks. I do not even want to be the team getting talked at by upper management when FDA investigators leave. I always felt compassion for the firm, but my hope was the learning experience I tried to provide them with. This is not just about what you did wrong but a chance to pick up and course-correct for regulatory compliance. The center team members did not like to advise the inspected firms of best-case course correction and many times deferred to the available guidance. I tried to sneak in some hints or nods or anything to acknowledge the proposed corrections were in the right direction. I gave no quarter to firms committing outright fraud or cooking the books. If a firm's employees caused the issues without management direction, then that is a different case study. I have twelve years of FDA regulatory experience that wants to flood you with knowledge, but it would come out garbled and complex. Let's build the foundation and establish trust with verification.

Industry closeout meetings for bioequivalence inspections with issuance of a 483 form always ended with the request for more FDA BIMO guidance. The look on the team's face every time this question is posed is priceless. I feel just like industry does, and I feel FDA should give updated detail-oriented guidance for bioequivalence. The molecular level is not an easy environment to work in. The global bioequivalence industry is hungry for more direction and expectation from FDA. Industry gets one or two chances a year to hear from FDA directors about bioequivalence guidance. The center should loosen the reigns of the field staff, but I understand the need to meet with the group to discuss pros and cons.

The FDA DSI center staff must meet with each other after an inspection and then the inspected firm get a meeting with the DSI center contact. I will advise firms to be patient with the DSI review staff they send all over the country and world. If it takes too long to get the review team together to put guidance out, then let them give preliminary thought process. In my opinion FDA should try not to make firms sweat out the inevitable decision of unacceptable work that will not be approved. The bioequivalence field of industry is getting tight with corporate giants dominating the international market. The hostile environment for start-up bioequivalence firms in the United States discourages even the most motivated individuals. Most big- and medium-size pharmaceutical companies demand regulatory compliance and reproducibility for every health care project.

My biggest FDA cases with wide-reaching regulatory implications came from bioequivalence inspections. Some of my cases spanned five years with hundreds of affected test articles and protocols. I had to get creative with the amount of exhibits I collected. The district was overwhelmed with the amount of documentation collected and the possible expense to ship the documents to the district and center. I was able to submit an electronic exhibit on multiple CDs.

I can tell you with a straight face, FDA investigators do not wish for the big case simply because of the mountain of work to document the case. I wished for compliant customers dedicated to patient safety and protocol compliance. You cannot wish for a better customer than the one I just described. I hope all of you out there conducting this very important business understand the global applications to your projects. Remember, we will all at one point need health care, so do your best every day to make a positive impact on our small world.

Institutional review boards (IRBs)/ethics committees and Radioactive Drug Research Committee (RDRC) were top BIMO priorities during my FDA tenure. I learned more about the FDA BIMO program from conducting IRB audits than in any training offered by the agency. IRB audits encompass a full range of the BIMO program and, in many cases, cover multiple departments within a hospital system. I was fortunate to inspect some of the most prestigious IRBs and hospital-system ethics boards with world-renowned staff. My first big warning-letter cases came from an IRB inspection audit with 483 observations that escalated to regulatory compliance actions. I started to review at least six protocols minimum for every IRB audit around 2005. I reviewed above and beyond what the CPGM or center-directed assignment requested. The way I looked at it was if an IRB is reviewing and approving over one hundred human clinical trials, I was going to spend no less than a week to ensure compliance. The FDA guide requires that field investigators review at least four FDA-regulated clinical trials. I would focus my review on high-risk-device protocols and vulnerable-population studies. Many of my big cases involved device-approval violations and unapproved drugs used in IRB approved clinical trials. I had a hard time understanding how IRBs did not ensure FDA approval before granting IRB approval. The first thing I would ask a principal Investigator seeking IRB approval for a clinical trial is for FDA application acknowledgment documentation (NDA, IND, PMA, 510K, etc.).

I have inspected some of the largest and smallest central/hospital-system IRB operations in the Dallas District. Both of my biggest cases were on cancer health providers and are the first cases that come up when you search my name, comma FDA. My first big IRB inspection came very early in my career when I was asked to inspect one of the biggest hot potatoes in FDA history. The FDA had litigated a case for twelve years and came out on the short end of the outcome. The centers were politically apprehensive to regulate this Houston based private IRB. The strategy was to regulate the Clinical Investigator through their IRB approval system. The process took ten years to finally get regulatory results. The first time I issued this IRB a lengthy 483 observation form, the center classified the result as no action indicated. The 483 form I issued listed observations that violate every major regulation IRBs have. I was disappointed and frustrated that so much hard work and detail on my first big case were wasted. I will state that historically FDA always recommends at least voluntary action indicated (VAI) anytime a 483 observation form is issued (unless 483 is flawed or not of regulatory concern).

Three or four years later, I was tasked with going back to this IRB for inspection. As before, the IRB had strayed from the regulatory path plus it had approved various test articles that had been placed on FDA hold. I documented most of the major violations and hoped the center would not fail me yet again. It took a year for the center to decide on the official-action-indicated classification with a warning letter.

During the yearlong waiting time, my district quality auditor reviewed my report and decided that I had not done a good job documenting my evidence. I was written up for not including key violations and documenting IRB member responsibility. I could not understand how such good work product could be second-guessed and documented as below standard. I pointed out to the auditor that all the items I was missing in the report were in fact in the report and detailed every page my information could be found. It was somehow my fault the center did not put an action forward. The following month, the center congratulated me on my report and the warning-letter issuance. The quality auditor amended their report to show I did a great job. The Dallas District never recognized my compliance work on this case or the ten years I spent trying to restore FDA's image. This case will never go away because politics and Hollywood rally behind so-called victims of FDA regulatory abuse. I say if your test article is biostatistically less effective than a placebo/sugar pill, it's time to find an effective therapy. If more patients expire in your human clinical trial than are held in remission/cured, then your hypothesis has failed scientific method. You cannot wish for a chemical entity to cure all forms of cancer. The best we can do right now is get your body cells to recognize cancer as foreign tissue before the cancer spreads to multiple tissues. There have been great strides in turning on the cell death cycle so the cancer cells do not live forever but harmlessly die as programmed.

I do not seek recognition for any of my accomplishments. I was happy to just protect and serve the unsuspecting cancer patient, giving away their life savings to the very end. If your product is found to be effective and safe for use in the most sick among us, then prove it. We will all have some form of cancer during our short lives here on earth. The very sun that makes life possible also sends harmful rays that ensure cancer will affect all of us.

The next giant IRB case I had come very early in my career as well. We were recognized by the district back then for this one because the firm is world renowned for excellence in cancer therapy. The inspection team went to the IRB and the Radioactive Drug Research Committee (RDRC). We found multiple violations and issued 483 observations forms that resulted in warning letters. The goal is not to get as many regulatory actions as possible; the goal is to document every case like it is going to be considered for FDA legal action. The compliance legal teams have the final say in whether a case is good enough to be tested in federal court. Both of the firms immediately implemented corrective action with no further action necessary.

I was thrown into the big FDA world after both of these high-profile cases. I would say that most of my work in Houston, TX was high profile. The professional clinicians I worked with were world renowned for their hard work and effective treatments. I still receive contact from this firm and will always work with them to fight cancer. I respect the effective work this firm does and have even sent family members with cancer to them for treatment. It is very difficult to take on thousands of clinical trials and keep track of every detail. The FDA really should foster a strong team-based approach to IRB regulatory compliance. The FDA reaches across the aisle for sponsors and test-article manufacturers, but the IRBs get a sort of mild neglect approach.

I will continue to believe that IRBs are a key component to ensuring patient safety and clinical-trial regulatory compliance. The IRBs in regulatory compliance should understand the protection they provide is vital to the FDA. The IRBs will regulate and review more human clinical trials than the FDA ever will. The FDA will always have the final approval for market authority. The FDA BIMO program will sadly review less than 1 percent of the human clinical trials ongoing in the United States and the world. I suggested many times throughout this book that FDA should conduct more BIMO inspections. FDA does not need more funds from taxpayers. FDA needs to utilize every penny of taxpayers' dollars like gold.

There will be waste in every organization, and the bell curve always applies. IRBs will have to be tolerant of the mild neglect and get ready for more oversight from more government agencies. Bioethics and human clinical trials will be an upcoming focus area for all domestic IRBs. The FDA centers are documenting which IRBs have bioethics discussions and ethics members on the review board. IRBs are not mandated to have ethics staff members on staff. I will not be surprised if the new CPGM and CFRs mandate IRBs to have ethics committee members. Many changes are on the way as more oversight agencies get involved with this process. I will personally always want to work with IRBs because I believe in the work they do. I want to help review boards conduct as many QA audits on their current approved clinical trials. I want to help bridge the small gap between IRBs and the FDA. I also want to help IRBs understand the great responsibility their members have in reviewing and approving human clinical trials.

In this world, humans and life forms in general must adapt to the environment for survival or perish. The FDA, in general, is very slow to adapt to the changing market environment. I stated before and will say it again; FDA is a reactionary force when a proactive approach is necessary. The centers are trying to put out fire and fight off regulatory noncompliance. It may not be enough to simply state to firms; I want all the data points and every scenario plausible. Scientifically based work is not intuitive, and it follows a plan. Guidance should not be used as a way to put in more regulation. Guidance should be a means to accomplish regulatory compliance without guesswork. The problem with good guidance is that it takes time to draft and review (work). Yes, FDA center staff, it takes real hard work, the work that has been put off for too long. "Do what I say, not what I do" is not going to motivate big business regulatory compliance in 2014 or beyond.

Get the FDA house in order and get to *work*! It is almost like I am telling FDA centers the same thing I am telling Clinical Investigators. Make sure you can accomplish the mission before you just send out a one-person army to do the job of ten individuals. The center needs to make sure the troops/field investigators are not spread too thinly or multitasking, to the point of not accomplishing anything. I would not be writing this book if FDA was accomplishing even 30 percent of the work. Conducting twenty or thirty BIMO inspections should not be considered impossible or unnecessary. Many of the upper management within FDA speak about the great accomplishments FDA has made. I would like to ask them; just when did accomplishing less than 1 percent of the total work became a great accomplishment?

Most of the BIMO investigators I know accomplish ten or fifteen inspections mixed in with non-BIMO work. At this rate, the BIMO work will truly not get above 1 percent. I have witnessed many BIMO investigators pride themselves on how long it took to complete their no-action-indicated inspection. It does not take three weeks at a firm to conclude no 483 is necessary. This is a direct burden to the firm and FDA. I have completed a multisite trial review with same amount of study subjects in Houston and Los Angeles district in half the time. It took me four days to complete my twenty-seven-subject review, with complete review of all subjects and documents. It took the LA investigator two weeks to conduct the same protocol inspection with no 483 form issued. This is a test case for FDA certification for BIMO field investigators. If industry must prove individuals are qualified and proficiently trained to conduct their business, then so should the FDA. FDA has left cleaning up its own house in favor of global oversight and posturing for some big dance. This is not a dance, and the business must not be farmed off to countries that do not have robust, effective environmental and patient-safety controls. The United States has a very difficult time ensuring our environment is safe, and we fail miserably at cleaning up superfund sites, Gulf of Mexico oil spill; and the list goes on. FDA will have to continue trusting but verifying globally. FDA's budget will decrease over the long run for lack of available no borrowed funds or civil will to increase the funding. FDA has to share funding among all the Health and Human Service branches (EPA, USDA, CDC, and other agencies programs).

The focus for the regulatory landscape will be enhanced inspections with an emphasis on encouraging and mandating all electronic records. The e-records review process will have to be hammered into the new field investigators. The new team will have to learn very quickly how to reverse engineer complex e-system and to apply rudimentary knowledge in order to understand industry innovation. As stated earlier, partner governments will have to implement environmental regulations and full product-cycle oversight. The time it will take to train partner-government inspectors and get industry to a level of compliance will take years, not months. You cannot simply send your standards or replicate a system by providing just the framework. You need the domestic industry base in the right mind-set and on your team. This is a team effort, but motivation is as unique as the amount of languages that are spoken on this planet. Mountains of cash will be required for outfitting functional electronic systems for global partner agencies. How will we pay for this grand global effort? Economics prohibit some of this universalization of global health when the focus must remain domestic. Keep it simple Sam (KISS). The government should learn from industry innovation and a shrewd cost prospective.

It does not always seem like the FDA mission comes first. It would appear to the field investigator that what matters to upper management is political gain and name recognition. I propose that you FDA managers conduct business effectively and efficiently with the public health in mind, you will be recognized for those efforts. Let's move forward to one of the most important aspects of the current modernization efforts globally that is enhanced electronic-systems review. Industry has waited more than a decade for guidance on 21 CFR Part 11.

CHAPTER 7

Electronic-Records Review

IN 2000, I received forty hours of computer validation training by the agency. It has been a long on-the-job-training road to where the global health industry is right now. Field investigators since 2001 have been requested to review regulated industry's computer systems. The FDA's infrastructure technology for the field has been slowly adapting yet always a step behind what is necessary to review computer systems. I had three laptop computers and one desktop personal computer in my twelve-year FDA career. Most of my industry peers have had computer refreshes at least every three years. I have had to deal with the slowest, most-frustrating computer systems in the world of global health. I cannot tell you how much time I wasted simply turning on my computer. Getting the many clunky software systems FDA installs on new hardware to work was also federal project. The amount of waste from cloning computers with different operating systems or versions of legacy software into a brand-new computer will always puzzle me. The grand scheme of things is such that waste in man-hours and sanity is ingrained in government computer technology.

I have sat idle for hundreds of hours waiting for my GOV business computer to decide whether to operate over twelve years. Most of the software systems routinely locked themselves up over my decade-long career. The main field accomplishments and compliance tracking system (FACTS) would slow to a snail pace or crash at the end of each fiscal year. Field investigators rush to in-put accomplishment hours and request endorsement approval through the FACTS system. I have also had waited for hours/days on software system repairs due to a centralized computer-tech hub system. Working from remote locations has been a blessing for staff but a security nightmare for government and industry alike. Much of the billions in government electronic system waste should be a focus area for all agencies (asset, e-waste, and hardware). The mountains of wasted taxpayer dollars in computing infrastructure are traceable. The GAO and HHS OIG will have a target-rich citation environment when it comes to E-Systems waste. FDA should mandate strict requirements for procuring E-Systems hardware and software. You have to wonder what upper management was thinking, procuring these clunky systems that routinely lock up or bug out. Were the decisions to procure FDA software systems based on future application of needs or politics and lowest bidder? Computer-system training for the field investigators has been much like the computer-system procurement system.

I have lost more data from software failure and hardware crashes that you begin to wonder if they purposely give you faulty equipment just to watch you go crazy. I have had to go outside just to blow my fuse at the waste of time and life force while dealing with the most convoluted e-system I have ever had to endure. The FDA will have to modernize every software system and hardware system every three years to keep up, and that will just not happen. The fair and open contract system for procuring new computer systems prohibit quick decisions; and the FDA, in general, will make what it has work even if it's snail speed. I have to tell my children, you get what you get and you don't throw a fit. I was told the same thing many times by the district IT department when I tried to explain that I needed a new laptop over a four-year period.

I had statements on record documenting the many FDA computer-system failures and wasted time because you cannot do anything without your machine. I cannot express the amount of frustration I felt trying to be proactive and efficient. I cannot get paid and sit idle, and many of my fellow government workers did just that on a regular basis. This job is too important to be allowing waste and precious time lost due to government's dinosaur procurement issues. When you crush efficiency, you crush your output and the willingness to succeed in the mission.

All of us new hires were trained and requested to review computer records from about 2001 onward. Over the years, I was trained in computer systems validation bit-by-bit, program area by program area. My official training record for computer systems lists two validation classes for a grand total of eighty hours. This is misleading because every training held for the drugs, devices, biologics, and BIMO programs incorporated computer-system validation and review. I will state for the record that most of my training was accomplished on the job. Many of the bioequivalence inspections offered a chance for me to work side by side with field experts from the Division of Scientific Investigations (DSI).

For the BIMO program, many computer-systems review approaches are overlapping; however, some, like in the bioequivalence program area, are uniquely complex. I routinely requested bioequivalence firms to provide me with all regulated computer-system documents and knowledgeable staff to explain them in depth. From very early in my career, the e-records revolution has exponentially entered every facet of our daily lives. We are desperately tied to our machines and helper robots to function in this business. The goal is to ensure the machines and software we rely on are consistently accurate with documented reproducibility. Validating compliant E-Systems takes man-hours, a technical skill set, and assets. FDA is now requiring field investigators to review critical E-Systems on every inspection. Get ready; your wait is over. The inspection requirements have been around for a decade, and it's time to check under the hood of your E-Systems (electronic).

FDA management and the current White House administration are mandating a paperless government, which is a great cost-saving effort. Sounds like a great catchphrase although the paper-reduction act is from 1995. There will always be a need for paper documentation as a security blanket to the elders. The many problems that come with paper storage and maintenance may outweigh the cost benefits. In our current time of big weather, I have gone in to cities after three hurricanes, and the logic for paper-only records becomes counterproductive. I have observed human clinical research firms that have lost all their paper-only documents in floods, tornadoes, and other natural disasters. It is very costly to redo a human clinical trial, and that cost goes up every year. Our field, domestic, and import FDA offices in Houston were flooded from top to bottom. FDA lost many historical paper-only documents due to water and mold damage. In 1998, we still did some triplicate carbon manual typing and other manually typed reporting (paper-based system). I started with FDA just when the manual typewriter was replaced with desktop computers.

The FDA is slowly making its way into the twenty-first century. There will always be a case for paper and against it, but that is for another book. I would only hope that our fresh drinking water and natural resources would be the focus for all discussion on the need for paper records. Recycled paper is great and should be used, but paperless systems do not use a drop of freshwater to make. If they could use seawater to make paper, then go for it; we have plenty of ocean water. Clean drinking water is becoming scarce, and climate change is flooding some areas out. My point is that it takes too much water to produce a roll of paper. I will always try to balance progress with sustainable and renewable ways when discussing any business-modernization platform. The fact is, if businesses do not think about a sustainable future and low-environmental-impact business models, there will be nothing left for our future generations. Do you really want to put yourself out of business because of overconsumption and gross environmental mismanagement?

We live in a delicate balance, and nature reminds us how toxic we are to our green biosphere. We only have one earth, which is shared by billions of creatures, and only ourselves to blame.

The FDA standardized the report content and writing for regulated industry around 2002. I was in Dallas, September 11, 2001, in Turbo electronic inspection record (EIR) training. The Turbo EIR system is the current standard for FDA. An updated system may be implemented, called the Mission Accomplishment and Regulatory Compliance Services system (MARCS) will take over (FACTS plus an import interface). The web-based TURBO EIR and FACTS systems are currently functional; however, many times, final field reports do not seem to populate or make it into the web-based system. The import division uses the Operational & Administrative system Import Support (OASIS). The OASIS system is anything but a beautiful tropical island worth visiting. I thankfully did not have to train on or use the OASIS system, but I did see it lock-up in action many times. When domestic field investigators collect certain types of samples the OASIS system must be accessed. I always picked one of my import buddies to help me with this task. No system is perfect, and some are less than desirable. The constant software patches and fixes seem to indicate the current reporting system is overwhelmed by the world of information that is FDA. I do not miss the computer systems FDA had us using or the centralized hardware/software technical-support system. Let's get back to training and review programs from around 2004 to 2011.

Regulated industry has been requesting electronic-systems guidance for many years with minimal response from FDA. The European model is much further ahead in the update and modernization aspect of electronic systems review. The focus has been on validation implementation, risk analysis of critical systems, data security, data integrity, communication, quality assurance, reproducibility, and compliance with 21 CFR Part 11. I will expand on each mentioned focus area, which again is only scratching the surface of the E-Systems world. I may leave you with more questions than answers, and that is the FDA way. Your electronic systems should be based on paper equivalence. This is of course easier said than accomplished.

Electronic systems are very complicated and costly to maintain in an effort to replace the paper system. When I received questions during an FDA-regulated inspection about electronic systems, I would base my response on the paper model. If you expand the paper model to the electronic model, you will get logical results.

Validations for hardware and software are critical starting points for any electronic system. When companies let the accountants decide how robust validations should be, field investigators line the 483 observation items up for you and the world to see. I would recommend logical science-based validation for your software and hardware systems because a robust system will pay for itself quickly. Your reward will be no 483 observations for quick and dirty validations. The center experts are well versed in all the shortcuts and cookbook failures. The advantage of being in the regulator seat is exposure to every test case multiple times over. As a quality assurance consultant, I will now have to recommend, advise, and hope for the best. I cannot tell the future, nor do I have a crystal ball, and the FDA field investigator will decide. I do know what is expected of your systems and how to ensure that when your friendly field investigator leaves, you will be happy. Validation is a cradle to grave evolving process with documented QA and maintenance. You do not just validate a system/an equipment and decide, "OK, great job, we're done." Your entire operation is expecting your systems to stay online, reproducible, secure, and maintained. This will take up the lion's share of your costs because it is your base. When mistakes are measured in recalls and adverse events/lives lost, tolerance for error is very low. Multimillion-dollar legal problems and brand-wrecking media coverage are the last things companies need in this economically challenged world.

Validation requires different reporting and maintenance for each program area. I will provide BIMO, biologics, and drug validation processes. I did not conduct device-manufacturer inspections, but I used to manufacture in vitro devices. I have conducted over a hundred device BIMO inspections. TradeStone QA has former FDA device field inspectors on the team. The FDA device program area also needs an inside scoop manuscript. The issues with FDA district device specialist turnover and slow guidance are never ending.

The BIMO program does not have a separate training program for validation and relies on the Center for Drug program. The Center for Biologics has a training program for validation mixed with the advanced biologics training, which I received. The validation approach for the drug and biologic programs are similar in nature with complementing and overlapping guides. The BIMO-validation program area encompasses all the centers except food. I have left the Center for Veterinary Medicine out in much of this book, but it is a very important program area that I have worked in my entire career. I have conducted veterinary drug and BIMO inspections. If any of the firms I inspected had computer systems, I routinely checked under the hood. I went above and beyond program expectations because every inspection is tied to a loved one, no matter if it's your mom or family pet. Our livestock for food production are also in this program area, CVM is vital for domestic health.

The basic validation standards were presented to us in the Good Automated Manufacturing Practice (GAMP) model. The ICH/EMA model has not been fully implemented into the FDA training programs. The basic principles between process validation and automated systems validation each have unique criteria for implementation. The focus is to determine if your operation has identified significant processes that require validation. The 21 CFR parts 211 and 11 apply to validation-process procedures for drug manufacturing. BIMO, as I stated before, is included in the drug-manufacturing control with the biologics regulation overlapping. Electronic systems are composed of many parts networked together by hardwire or wireless link. The full range of electronic systems must be validated for use in manufacturing or human clinical research. The risk-based approach is the current model and works for now. Emerging technology may mitigate the minutia involved with proving your network is change controlled, secure, and maintained by intelligent design. If you build a system with compliance and performance from the ground up by intelligent design, your output will be market ready!

Data-management life cycle, coding, integration, and software development were left out for on-the-job training. It is difficult to complete a mission with half the skill sets necessary, but you do what you can with what you have. I have done a lot of homework after eight hours at the site, looking up things in the FDA e-library I knew nothing about. The installation and operational and performance-qualification system were drilled into us (IQ, OQ, PQ). I was not ready for the mountain of notebooks that was brought before me, detailing the validation master plan, final report, and maintenance documentation. Only the IT workers and management know about the volume of paper reams in binders or thousands of pages on a file format. I have been asked many times if I was sure they had to bring all the binders. My answer was always yes and then I got to work. Then the next surprised look was when I found the system failures or out-of-specification result with no documented investigation. It is good to be underestimated because then you have the upper hand. Familiarization with Chess, Texas hold'em poker, and chicken should be – required for FDA field investigators. These life games may be used to prepare the new hires for the global health mission.

Consider what it takes to train anyone in computer-systems validation for bioequivalence (clinical and laboratory), GMP, cGMP, GLP (nonclinical and clinical), GCP, and ICH. Then consider more than half the training is on the job in the field; figure it out or go home crying. I have seen a few field investigators ball up and freak out after a few days with me in the field. It takes a can-do, never-give-up constitution to stare down the mountain of data and say, "Yes, I climbed Mount E-data Systems today and survived." The building blocks and basic training approach are two ways to operate with college-level team members. The risk-based approach peels away the layers to get to the focus area that you then have to branch from. You must review a fair sampling of the validation material or risk not finding the needle in a haystack. The main regulatory approach is also focused on your company's failures or whatever word you use to describe out of specification, nonconformance, change control, reject, and recall. The field investigator will root out your procedures and failures to connect the dots. In essence, your health firms have trained me to conduct computer systems suitability audits because by going through the stacks, you stumble upon knowledge. I cannot tell you how much beginner's luck plays for the prepared mind during a systems validation review. Many times, IT personnel stumble upon the system failures by reviewing them with me or explaining them to me, and the light bulb goes on for both of us. Do not use luck in trying to validate your systems; leave that to the guys in funny green suits at the end of a rainbow.

Data security is of vital interest to your validated systems and equipment. In the age of hackers, international theft of intellectual knowledge and government snooping, security is mandatory. How many layers of security and how you train your employees dictate how secure your systems are. You obviously want to start with a compliant system. Physical and logical controls secure access portals. Access levels for the operator, supervisor, engineer, and administrator. Audit trails for an access point are vital to ensure the data-stream integrity. Cloud-based computing has taken over online storage processes, and offline data backup should be included in your security protocol. Source code security and access controls should be robust, or your entire infrastructure will be vulnerable. System- and platform-level security procedures should have qualification and consistent review. Layering access for change control and the ability to disable access are key requirements. Backup archives and recovery systems are part of the security process. Let's move to your weakest links or your best defense, which are employee passwords and online access points.

Employee passwords and remote access points are the most vulnerable parts of your e-system. Both of these portal points are out of your control and your responsibility at the same time. Training your team about using secure-access wired and wireless Internet portals should be the first step. Auditing your remote-access supplier and challenging your systems security should be part of the process. You may even want to get one of your IT staff or hack consultants to hack in or attack your system. Internet-security firms specialize in challenging your system. This may be something to consider for a regular protocol challenge. E-Systems should have intrusion detection and shutdown or defensive reactions.

If the CIA system can be hacked, does anyone out there stand a chance? It is becoming very clear that system security needs to be rethought. Security is not just a word; it is a process of managing your company and the intellectual knowledge built from the ground up. Make sure your system infrastructure is not secure in word only. The FDA mandates of electronic submission just revealed new problems to securing data streams. Paper is easily defended in a vault, slowly deteriorating but in your control. IT gurus, make sure your companies' active and passive e-security controls are in place. In some cases, your customers may not even know they are being hacked. Online and offline enhanced security systems will make up the difference between profits and losses. There are no shortcuts for this process.

Data integrity seems like a simple-enough statement until you implement your proposed plan and realize the complexity. There are three modes of constraints for integrity; these are entity, referential, and domain when integrated for a relational data-model. Source-data capture for clinical trials, data movement within the system, metadata/audit trails, and review of data are vital aspects to the data integrity, ensuring your critical-data systems/ E-Systems are certified consistent and reconcilable with respect to output or data review. Progressive quality assurance for database integrity will ensure accuracy in the represented data. I have lost some of you, and that is OK because we are not all IT minded. Some of you are thinking that I have over-simplified the IT section and that is ok as well. I am not writing an IT manual the world is full of them. These concepts are so basic and simple that they, inherently, are overanalyzed for complexity.

Think of it in terms of your paper-based model. You generate written or typed data in printout form. You check your data points for accuracy, and QA or monitors review the data. Printout documentation must be stored in a secure environment, safe from deterioration or manipulation for future regulatory review or application approval. Data integrity is this basic paper/analog concept in the digital environment. The predicate rule to 21 CFR Part 11 contains the description and definition of this concept. Does Part 11 need to be updated and expanded? Most of the IT industry experts I speak with are tired of waiting and frustrated with the lack of clear, plain language not open for multiple interpretations. Is the FDA going toward the EMA/ICH models of computer-system regulatory oversight? All the centers with e-system program areas will have to be included in any guidance generated by FDA.

Network communication via wired or wireless access points is the nerve center to your E-Systems. Without controlled and interruption-free network communication, your products will not make it to market. Network communication must have security controls and traceability to ensure data integrity. Most, if not all, of your integrated systems will be fair game for FDA review unless you have something to hide. When I was told no by a firm that I could not review "internal audit" documentation, the outcome was always yes. I have observed that most firms deem internal audits as failure investigations or deviations they find during routine review. This information is within FDA scope of review unless it deals with corporate-accounting monetary figures. Companies must understand field investigators must assure that you are following your procedures and the 21 CFR regulations. FDA interpretation of regulated documentation and industries must meet at the conjunction of understanding. In plain language, do you want a refusal noted on your inspection and a production hold or warning letter? Do not hide your violations; a good investigator will find the problems with or without your help. If your company is transparent with corrective actions and investigation process, you have self-compliance, which is the goal to strive for. Your standard operating procedures must be verified and documented for review. How do you expect FDA investigators to verify your investigational procedures without reviewing "internal documents"? When a customer or vendor asks you for this information, you gladly comply because money is on the table. Well, think of it the same way with FDA. Your production or process is on the table when FDA investigators audit your firm. You can either comply or receive a 483 observation form with a warning letter to follow. Your brand will be affected, and your customers may seek more-compliant competitors. This is not a shell game of how to hide the violations. I have had the frustrating task of investigating many firms trying to sweep violations under the rug in the hopes I would not see the observations. I do not play games, and I always found the violations by review design or pure luck. You can follow the trail of 483 observation forms I have issued to verify my statements. I am not the best, and I am not the worst FDA investigator, but I always did my best to protect and serve you all. If you have public health at heart and a good knowledge base, success is the only option.

Network-communication review and 21 CFR Part 11 compliance should be incorporated into any e-system your company builds or acquires. Your networks are critical and should be designed with regulatory compliance from the ground up. Build quality into your entire operation for market-ready products and compliant clinical trials. I am not trying to train you or give you an all-inclusive overview. I am starting at the high level of E-Systems regulatory requirements for your base-building concepts. Triple-check your e-system regulatory compliance so that when FDA inspects your operations, there are no surprises at the conclusion of the visit.

Quality assurance of your E-Systems should be on a scheduled, logic-based interval. Ensuring reproducibility in your e-system with documented audit-based procedures is a logic-based approach. If you have to ask the accountants every time you need to ensure quality-based systems are installed, you better get it right the first or second time around. I will stay in the recommendation mode when speaking with your upper management with a twist of regulator insight for good measure. You will find that I can be very persuasive without any push. I find that reality and documented regulatory evidence will loosen the shrewdest decision maker. I can guarantee my statements and history of documented results with respect to my experience. I have lived in the public eye under strict conduct principles mandated by FDA service. Every action you make in public service is closely monitored by your handlers and the unknowns (internal affairs). I have held to a high moral and ethical standard that many of you can relate to. Honor and integrity have been forged into my heart and mind. Of course, I slip up and fall down, but I have not crashed and burned. I have not cut any corners or taken any manila envelopes under the table because saving lives is priceless.

I have already discussed with you the vital aspect of QA at every significant and critical process, but consider the EMA model for a moment. Are third-party QA auditors routinely putting another set of eyes on your process for ensured and continued success? Why not? What are you afraid of, some scammer taking you for a ride? Of course you are. Qualify your third-party QA, check the references or just call my team; I worked for the guys that are coming to visit your firm. My systematic approach will vaccinate your whole organization for the mean big blue regulators. I have only skimmed the world of E-Systems; the real detail will come when my team is working on enhancing your entire operation.

Inspection approach and compliance with 21 CFR Part 11 are industries' million-dollar questions. FDA is now mandating more electronic application submission for medical health products and all electronic medical records. The FDA needs to abide by these initiatives and show industry how to accomplish this all-electronic model. Lead by example and industry will recognize the inherent guidance of a successful model. I continue to field questions from industry regarding computer-systems review. Many industry managers do not believe me when I say the FDA is now reviewing and documenting E-Systems compliance with ICH and 21 CFR Part 11. It almost seems like I am speaking a different language to them because I almost have to convince them that I am not trying to drum up QA business. After a decade of waiting, many of you in the industry have allowed your systems to fall out of compliance or never started with compliant systems. Retroactively patching a system to comply with regulations puts your fragile network in jeopardy to fail challenges by the experts. It may be time to seek a model with all the basic requirements or pay triple in the long run for failure. Software, hardware, firmware, and auxiliary network devices have a limited life cycle that cannot be changed.

Made in anywhere but USA does not last the entire life of your company. You cannot expect to get ten times of what you paid for your systems; get over it. It is like your automobile tires or brakes; they were made to last a certain life cycle so you can go back and buy again or find a tailored model. I have many IT professionals ready to review and recommend best-fit model or how to get the most out of your current compliant model.

The field-inspection approach will always start from the highest level of your E-Systems in a stepwise approach to the bottom with all the milestone stops along the way. The first steps include determining if your firm has identified critical and significant processes in your e-system. The second step is validation documentation review and a demonstration of performance. The third step will be to request your failures in whatever term you use to define out of specification or deviations. The list goes on, including the question, did you follow your investigation procedures or change controls? What is your security model and how do you ensure passive/active intrusion. What are your defensive controls if you have any? Training and ensuring employee adherence to the procedures and regulations can be a target-rich environment for failure if your QA is not enhanced. You do not have to work hard all the time, but you do have to be knowledgeable.

The cloud and other technologies will propel every one of us into new frontiers of public health care. The quantum computer and intelligent swarm servers will make gigabytes look like peanuts. The more our designs mimic nature, the more in touch we become with the natural environment. New materials for computing and production in the nanoscale will bring nanobots that heal and stay for a while or get passed on. The E-Systems you use now will seem like only a memory. Do not fall in love with your E-Systems because you will only be disappointed when it is time to break up the infatuation. Sail that puppy off and hold on tight because we are in the middle of a revolution that will elevate us to equal status like a family should be. Expect to use much of your empire's assets on E-Systems with light-speed life cycles because your whole operation depends on it.

CHAPTER 8

Regional/District Management Issues

SINCE THE REORGANIZATION effort started in 2006, there have been many proposals and modernization efforts to streamline the FDA groups/centers. Closing food- and drug-analysis laboratories were touted as a great way to cut cost. The measure may have been a ploy for more funds, but it made FDA look harebrained. The push to cut regional middle-management structure was a good idea that did not happen. Closing the laboratories for FDA would have been catastrophic. The fact is that FDA labs get overwhelmed with domestic/import samples and could use a few more modern labs for efficiency. I agree with cutting regional management because there are only a handful of them and they soak up high senior executive services (SES) monies. What does the region do for the field besides going to a meeting about the next meeting and counting beans for their big bonus? A computer program can count beans, and it does not want a bonus or fly business class. During my time at the FDA, I received fewer e-mails annually from the regional bosses combined than I have fingers on my hands. FDA needs more investigators, not bean counters, in my humble opinion.

I do not think the government should be the biggest spender of its own services; that is redundant waste (snail mail use). FDA mandates that industry go paperless. Well, shouldn't the FDA comply with a 1995 mandate? FDA should scan and send reports or use Turbo EIR for a web-based repository. If a FDA resident post needs the report, they just bring it up on the web as is current practice – a simple solution to paper and waste trails. The global public health needs the FDA in most cases. The FDA in turn needs to be more responsible with intellectual and physical resources.

The new FDA quality management system (QMS) and database tracking are currently stopgap measures slowing the already-slow work pace. I observed two speeds in my government service, which were slow and stop. I strived to accomplish the work of two individuals in that type of environment. It was very frustrating to complete an assignment ahead of schedule only to be stopped in limbo at the next stage of review. The supervisors are focusing on quality process and assignment requests multitasking with many other issues. The supervisors should be "chained to the desk," reviewing reports and getting work out. It appears the new supervisors are always in training and practicing "soft skills" instead of grinding out regulatory-worthy work product. Industry is the FDA's customer, and hopefully, regulatory compliance is the end product or outcome.

Personal-glory agendas have no place in public health or any professional organization. The district/regional/national levels of FDA are full of managers seeking political name recognition to go higher, who do not have public service as motive for the mission. It is not about how high you climb; it is about how many lives you save. I do not care about any of my national FDA awards or 483 observation forms with warning letters.

I care and want to know how many lives I have saved by conducting patient-safety-minded BIMO, drug, or biologics inspections. The reward is knowing you're not stepping on anyone or elevating yourself in your own mind, because no one is above another. We are equal with different jobs and pay grades. The solution is logical and simple, but you will not see it because you are blinded by ambition to become a legend in your own mind.

The current Dallas District management strategy is to promote individuals with seven or eight years of experience. These new supervisors have yet to prove themselves as good investigators and are now leading individuals with ten- and twenty-plus years in FDA service. Is this really a recipe for success? In any organization, it is best to have seasoned leaders with years of documented continuous success (not just one or two blips). I am not a businessman or even have much experience leading a team. We were taught to work as individuals and to think outside the box, but in the recent past, they tried to put us back in the box. The new way of training is to mold new field investigators into well-rounded generalists good at conducting any inspection. This is not practical or real-world application. The very managers that want generalists do not have enough FDA field experience or situational awareness that comes with many years of service (fifteen-plus years).

This generalist mentality will stifle retention and morale. The current workforce will struggle because each program area has many applications and regulated products. I have observed that professionals like to choose what program area they excel in, and they develop more skills as time goes on. There are no real jacks-of-all-trades for this job. If that is the case, then how does FDA expect to develop district or national specialists and experts?

The mission will be successful when management distributes the available skill sets appropriately throughout the district. Just to stay relevant and knowledgeable in one program area, the field investigator has to be on top of all current guidance and regulatory policy changes. The biologics program area changes quarterly, sometimes monthly; and if you do not stay relevant, mistakes will be made.

Each program has a multiversity of responsibilities. I like to think of it this way. The FDA should be the BDDF administration (the biologics, devices, drugs, and food administration), so the order of importance is listed alphabetically. I put biologics first because so many patients use blood products/tissue harvesting every day, and there is so much personalized medicine in use. The rest of this is intuitive for most of you out there. Food is important, and the fact that we have so many various layers of food agency protection that it should take a backseat ride. Does the United States really want affordable health care?

Innovation is required before affordability becomes part of the equation. Simply speaking, more clinical trials will have to be conducted in order for new innovative products to be approved. You cannot send a food investigator to conduct a device audit or BIMO inspection. Shift the landscape to foster innovation, not squash the market for who knows what reason. Focusing on tobacco and graphic art mandates are the showcase agendas for the political at heart. Food safety, including genetically modified organisms with irradiation processing, somehow seems to make big headlines. BDDF should be the focus in my dirt-level, humble opinion.

"Do more with less" is the mantra currently shouted by management; however, this only works if the grunts are compensated monetarily or with time off, including kudos for more great accomplishments. The FDA is far from doing anything but stepping on morale and requesting that investigators do the work of three people and stating, "At least you have a job, right?" Industries do get away with doing more with less because they give 10 or 15 percent bonus. Regulated industry has less workforce expenditures and manageable office overhead. The current performance evaluation system or PMAP is really an old system that was found to be subjective and unfair. The FDA managers brought it back to life after a decade of mothballs. It is difficult to find nice/professional words when describing this employee evaluation system. The FDA union has fought this change in rating systems and documented the subjective nature of the current evaluation system.

I recall one supervisor telling me that I would not get the highest possible rating because those were saved for the center or district management. The rating system is tied to an increase in pay so you can see how this would affect your annual pay and morale. I find it difficult to explain the glass ceiling I observed while enduring this subjective rating system. I was not compelled to produce more because; I am not a donkey trying to get a carrot dangling on a string from a stick. I knew I could not get the carrot and I did not move, end of story. Your reverse psychology is apparent and insulting. I did my best to consistently provide work-product above and beyond expectation. We expect to be given credit for doing more than we were asked to do. A simple email or word of gratitude will be sufficient, but an honest evaluation of the work product is required when dealing with professionals. My FDA colleagues knew when their supervisor was looking for every insignificant reason to give a bad review instead of detailing the mountains of good work.

The FDA really needs to cut down on paper use as in the Paper Reduction Act from 1995 and presidential mandates to recycle and be eco-friendly. FDA currently ships UPS and USPS daily for thousands upon hundreds of thousands of taxpayer dollars (snail mail, as we affectionately call our fellow civil servers). The FDA could save millions of dollars on reducing paper and paper-shipping cost in order to pass that savings on to the frontline investigators or the entire mission.

Here is a rhetorical Texas question: what happens when you try to stuff twenty pounds of cow manure in a five-pound paper sack? No, it's not a piñata unless you're an Aggie (I just had to; it is an inside Texas joke). The FDA investigator in the field does not do their job for recognition, fame, or glory. They do their job to protect and serve all of you with the knowledge their pay-rate is enough to just about make a decent living (most of the FDA crew I knew lived check to check). Contrary to public opinion, government workers are not overpaid for what they do; and yes, some civil servants may be considered jelly doughnuts (they are in every organization). Most of the Houston crew lived modest lives in average-size homes, nothing fancy. At the Houston cost-of-living adjustment, you might think, *Sweet deal,* until you see your gasoline receipts from driving in traffic for hours.

If FDA regional directors were able to improve employee moral with increased work product, they can stay, however this may never happen now the cat is out of the bag. You bigwig SES regional directors have only yourselves to blame for poor productivity and dissent in the ranks. There are too many grievances ongoing and in limbo with constant supervisor turnover. Full teams are pleading with upper management for change of duty station due to supervisory breakdowns and unqualified leadership. Time is wasting along with our FDA workforce. Top heavy towers with a shallow base will always fail.

Consumer safety officers (CSOs) or field investigators are behind the scenes and anonymous unless you request their reports or have received the dreaded 483 notice-of-inspection observation form and subsequent warning letter. CSOs do not take pleasure pointing out your firm's deficiencies because they know many times the result is management termination or possible further legal action. I will tell you that if your company has intentionally harmed the public by cutting corners for cost savings and falsifying records, there is no quarter for you when caught. FDA will expose your firm to the World Wide Web with a great big 483 spotlight (like the Batman light in the sky). In most cases, FDA is there to help you company correct your unintentional mistakes and steer your organization in the right direction.

FDA is not a consultant organization. FDA investigators consult on the regulations by issuing the 483 observation form. This 483 form is recommending that your firm operate within the 21 CFR regulations. The 483 list of observations form is FDA's interpretation of what regulations are most relevant to your operation.

A five-year pay freeze, doing more with less, and mismanagement will get you nothing more than red-eyed zombie-like civil servants. We can only hope that the individuals and upper management in charge read these recommendations for a proficient, effective FDA. *In the end, my management team wanted me to conduct blood-donor-center work; drug work, including CVM inspections; Seafood HACCP work; and maybe a little BIMO work.* My choices, which were per CSO position description for top three, were BIMO, drugs, and biologics.

I cannot be gone from home more than 50% of the time or be in two places at once. The BIMO prescription drug user fee act monies pay for almost half of the FDA staff's salary. Management wanted me to divert and dilute my drug auditing and BIMO skill sets. I was sent off to do wash out inspections and benched for grieving against the establishment. I had to relocate for my new young family's sake so that was my insubordinate crime for which I was benched. I wanted to stay in the BIMO field and that was not happening. This is one main reason, I regretfully left my post at FDA. I can tell you there is a world of BIMO work to be accomplished, so when I finish this book, its back to BIMO quality assurance and providing training to industry. This is my passion, and it motivates me to get up every morning and say, "Let's get in there and accomplish positive documented results." The FDA BIMO investigator field staff is a very small percent of the total workforce (at most 8 percent).

Update the BIMO program area, mandate certification, and utilize as much of your assets as possible; there is so much work to be done. Senior HHS leadership and FDA management, how are you going to provide an environment where vaccine manufacturers and drug pharma want to build domestically to secure adequate supply? The mainstream news media puts out many stories about medicine and vaccine shortages. How is it even possible that there can be any shortfall whatsoever in this country?

In the end, a perceived sense of safety is much more cost-effective than just a reliance on domestic self-compliance. I have asked higher ups, senior executive service (SES), why can't the FDA actually get to at least 50 percent of the human preclinical trials for data validation review? The answer was stated as follows, "Not all test articles will make it to market or be found effective and safe". I thought quietly to myself, "*Don't the patients in those studies on test articles that will not make it to market deserve an FDA review to ensure their patient safety?*" FDA can do more, and we all can do more to make regulatory compliance inherent to your operation. If you are in any way under FDA, ICH, EMU, regulations, we are in this global health struggle every day. We can innovate and meet the needs of our global health future.

I would just like to say it appears there are few FDA district management rattlesnakes to bag up and organize, which takes too much time. Choose responsible, seasoned management to run the system so that the only option is an efficient workforce. If the supervisor is delegated to perform the district investigator branch (DIB) functions, when do the inspection reports get reviewed and released? If the DIB is missing in action (MIA) and not conducting the mission, how does the rest of the district system function? There is no tolerance for failure at the DIB level. This is a high-level management position of leadership with team-building responsibilities. If your team is jumping ship, it may be that your ship is about to hit an iceberg and you will not listen to a recommended course correction.

Management gets caught up in the barking orders, not realizing how offensive they become. You do not become elevated; you are there to serve others, not to be served. If you want a good team effort, you have to roll your sleeves up and put your boots on for some real work. Managers, we know when you're delegating to save your own skin and we know when you're over your head. You have a duty to delegate to senior investigators for training purposes, but in small doses.

FDA investigators, the good ones, at least, can read individuals like a book; and your lack of experience is on the front page. Good leaders listen to the experts in the field and are willing to learn from a subordinate. Check your ego at the door management; the room is too small for all of us to fit in. There is a chain of command to follow, and it will always be that way. The military service is for rigid chains of command. FDA hires professional civil servants to become highly skilled in order to base observations with logic and science. We are not soldiers or war fighters that must do what they're told or die in the field. If a process or directive seems off the wall, most field investigators will recognize this right away. If you bark at me, I do not respond well to juvenile antics or the because-I-said-so mentality. Management's job is to ensure FDA provides a safe and secure work environment to the field.

Management is providing a pressure cooker due to micromanagement and second-guessing. Being in the field and conducting inspections are stressful enough; now you want to work me into a lather, no, thanks. You're not a parent or a friend; you're a work facilitator. Work gets assigned to your team; you make sure it gets distributed to the right inspectors and that it gets completed. When you supervisors get out reports and check for grammar and correctness, do not try to put your style in the report. You can make sure it flows or is coherent, but your flowery style will not make it into one of my reports ever. The BIMO-center review audience expects a certain caliber of report that does not include portions of the CPGM or why a requested exhibit was collected. If the CPGM mandates exhibits of certain information, it goes into the report with a brief sentence or list of observations.

The stopgap progress provides a festering sloth that creeps up on you. You start to wonder why a four-day inspection only takes three days to write and three weeks for your supervisor to review. Then you get the report back, dipped in red ink after ten years of dedicated, decorated service. The changes were style points or neat little descriptions of minutia that have no bearing on the content. If you want to write a neat report, get back in the field where you belong for some more seasoning. Supervisors get a substantial amount of training after they get the job. The new supervisors are gone for weeks, learning their new positions. It may be more effective to hire individuals that have gone through those training as investigators and on the job so that when they get in bingo, they get to work. Oh, this may take some time up front as an investigator, and that is the point. They need more time in grade learning all they can before leading seven or eight team members. There is no learning curve when you're leading a team because the mission cannot wait for you to catch up. It seems more logical to train a supervisor before you let them loose on seven or eight unsuspecting souls.

Transparency is a great buzzword until you find out how much guidance needs to be drafted and implemented for distribution in all program areas. The easy part is showing a database that is already in place, documenting the violations. What about the transparent guidance that is long overdue in the drugs, devices, BIMO, and biologics program areas? Regulated industry has been requesting center-directed guidance for ten years in the E-Systems.

The drug program area firms have so many new questions for FDA on chemistry manufacturing controls and the quality-by-design programs. The compliance program guide manual for radionuclide drug manufacturing has turned ten years old. FDA expects industry to get on track. Industry in turn may request that FDA get back on track and quit with the sidebar busy work. Meat and potatoes are on the menu FDA with no fluff. Politics should not mandate what this science-based organization must focus on. How can a decade go by without an FDA update that is almost an entire product life cycle? Industry has innovated and upgraded policies and procedures at least ten times in a decade.

Dedication and a sense of duty are only half of the management equation. Knowledge and wisdom are required for true leadership. A willingness to toe the line or get into the trenches must never fade from the frontline supervisor. The supervisors should be willing to step in and conduct some inspections to get the final numbers up. They should also stay relevant and not lose sight of the skills necessary for their employee's success. You cannot go soft and lukewarm as a manager! Your subordinates and team members will eat your lunch. I can smell a comfortably numb jelly doughnut from a mile away, and you know who you are (because you just scoffed). I want to encourage you to pick up the learning curve pace; the mission is waiting for all hands on deck. Is FDA really into the mission of protecting the public or is this just all for **Commerce Continuity (tax revenue).** Yes I did just say that!

I want to be your company's mentor, trainer, drill sergeant, and trusted colleague. This work we endeavor to accomplish is complex by nature and necessary for the health of our world. Your skill sets must be in this scientific work not strictly business because health care products are not just widgets. This health-care-product profession is an evolving life cycle of success and failure modes. Success is not measured in return on investment, for you gold miners or board of directors. Success is measured in lives saved and extended. Every life born to this earth has great potential to make a difference, good or bad. We each have free will to be enslaved or break the chains that bind us. We are bound by imagination alone and can change the landscape with a single brushstroke. There is no magic bullet for bacterial or viral infection, but that does not stop us from looking. Our bodies have the mechanisms to fight and recover from massive trauma and toxins when we live healthy. If the air we breathe and the water we drink are toxic, how can we extend our life cycles? If the land is contaminated with heavy metals, dioxin, and radionuclides, how many generations do you think we have left? Progress must continue, but not for the sake of progress alone. A sustainable future is one idea away from realization.

I do not wish for anyone at FDA to be demoted or terminated or even feel bad because of this manuscript. I have hope for every civil servant who takes the oath of public safety. I know the FDA will continue to promote public safety. The work will get accomplished and fresh faces will form the new upper ranks. The sink-or-swim method worked for my crop of newbies, and only time will tell how the recent influx of food-program inspectors works out. Management at the district level feels it is wise to hold back step increases with the already-imposed pay freeze. I do not see the wisdom in this thought process, but the troops are restless. These new hires are tomorrow's FDA leaders; do not crush them before the thirty-year time frame.

Let the slow progression of time march on with your stepwise approach, reinforcing the never-give-up team attitude. If you do not work as a team, you fail as an organization. Failure is not an option for FDA or any one of you working there. We can all succeed if we work together at this global challenge. The scientific method teaches us to learn from the mistake made along the way.

The roundtable-team approach will win the hearts and minds of the regulated industry. You may be surprised how many goals can be accomplished by simply discussing the viewpoints and compiling the visionary prospects. Let's have a cold fusion moment (light bulb). I would not be the same person I am without the one man and three women that were my supervisors at FDA.

I would like to have a beer/beverage summit with all my former teammates because twelve years is a long time to make friends. When I left the Houston resident post, they threw me a big (for FDA) lunch gathering with gifts and cards, as if I were going away for good (retiring). I was only going down the road to Austin for my young family's sake. I was moved by the family feel and well wishes from my FDA comrades. I will always cherish the good and bad. The FDA is my family, and it seems like I am the black sheep, but that could not be more false. I am for public safety and protection, so if that is what you work for, we work together. I may be somehow misguided or missing the boat, so fact-check me and challenge my recommendations scientifically. FDA business is not personal; it is a professional environment of producers and regulators.

I am an unknown/nobody, but at the same time, I am all of you because we are connected by a global health mission. We all matter; we all count as unique and equal individuals with free will. It is not a birthright or blood line that makes you great, nor is it the amount of money you die with. It is the example of service and leadership that makes mankind great. The folly of mankind is in our wish to be king or queen, not realizing that it is in the service of others that kings or queens are made. In a world of equals, there are no kings or queens, whom are above/elevated from anyone else. The current global struggle is for life without bondage or enslavement.

I also want to say to you, businesses that are leaving the United States, if you use slave labor to produce cheaper products, the market will know and reject your brand. The United States is full of capable and sharp-minded workers, ready for lifesaving jobs. I commend efforts to elevate third world countries, but have we diminished ours as a first world country in the process? Peace to all of you who seek peace and love. The rest of you can go to Mercury in peace or step across the aisle; we are waiting. Without passion for what drives mankind to achieve a perceived-impossible challenge, such as global health, our legacy will be lost in ashes.

It is a strange world we live in where the winner of the world's Peace Prize commands five wars and unknown amounts of kinetic actions every year in office. The First Lady has gotten into the global-health leadership mission by trying to keep children fit and health conscious. Follow your lady's lead, boss man. Let's focus on life while we still have it and leave death for natural causes. Liberty and justice for all! Let's focus on effective science-based global health care products and public safety in a team effort. We are not enemies or Texas hold'em players trying to one-up each other. We are the unknown guardians on a mission to ensure public health and safety. The word shortfall should not be used when speaking about the United States of America or public health.

Why did I leave my safe and secure public service job? I needed to work in a more-efficient and less-wasteful organization with science-based logic for a science-based environment. There will always be red tape and the need for accountability, but that is the beauty of electronic-based business. The bean counting is inherently done by the E-Systems in place, not political mismanagement. The small-business group and one-man armies will bring this country back from the brink of total annihilation. I have joined the private sector now to solve these grave global economic and health problems. Let's get to work, America, on innovation and products the world wants to buy. Stabilize the physical sustainable market and cyberspace for a future our grandkids can enjoy.

Fast forward three years now since this manuscript came to life. Tradestone QA has gone international two years in a row. Most of my clients are drug manufacturers and compound pharmacies in need of GMP audits for sterile and non-sterile products. My first thought was to add these two topics to this second edition however know it is apparent that a whole new book will have to be written. I will begin formulating this manuscript however it might be a while since we have been so busy attending to our clients. I appreciate your patience through this manuscript evolution. Connect with us on LinkedIn, follow us on Twitter or look us up online. Your comments and critiques help make this OUR project not just my project.

ACKNOWLEDGMENTS

I DEDICATE THIS book to the frontline FDA and ex-FDA investigators, support staff, laboratory staff, and the DSI Review Division; without your work and sacrifice, our country would not be as safe and our health products most effective. Without field investigators, there would be no center, region, laboratories, or management structure. Many senior managers have never served on the frontline nor can they lead by example. They do not know what it takes to really run the FDA show. Thank you to my colleagues, friends, and family for putting up with my antics and big head!

I would like to thank my professors at UTSA for giving me the technical base to build on in my career and exposing me to emerging biotechnology science. They said we were quacks for using fractal dimension calculations, and now fractal dimension is mainstream. To all the pioneer professors of biotech, I salute you. (Try, fail, and try again to succeed or fail again = the scientific method.)

IT help from Mr. Jorge Velazquez
J. D. Price collaborations
Kara Harrison, RAC, RQAP-GCP, *kara@qualityresearchconsultants.com My first FDA BIMO mentor*

If our TradeStone QA team can help improve your global health products in the regulatory life cycle to market, please contact us (*http://www. tradestoneqa.com/*) or link with US on LinkedIn (*http://www.linkedin.com/profile/view?id=67701210&locale=en_US&trk=tab_pro*).

INDEX

www.ingramcontent.com/pod-product-compliance
Lightning Source LLC
Chambersburg PA
CBHW031245280526
45784CB00004B/1731